PDQ
PrettyDarnedQuick

OTITIS EXTERNA

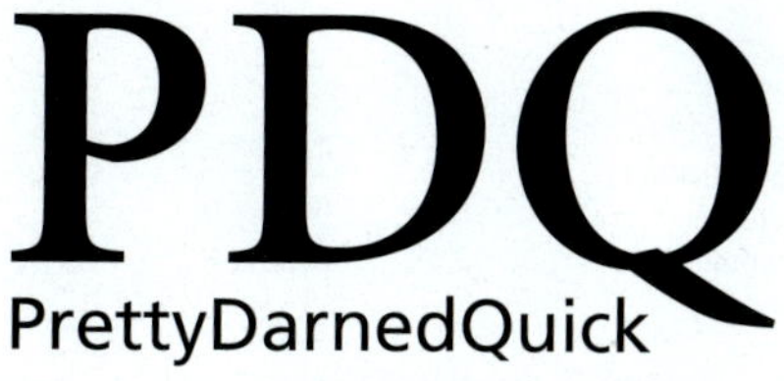

PDQ
PrettyDarnedQuick

OTITIS EXTERNA

Joseph Dohar, MD

2007

BC Decker Inc

Hamilton

BC Decker Inc
P.O. Box 620, L.C.D. 1
Hamilton, Ontario L8N 3K7
Tel: 905-522-7017; 800-568-7281
Fax: 905-522-7839; 888-311-4987
e-mail: info@bcdecker.com
website: www.bcdecker.com

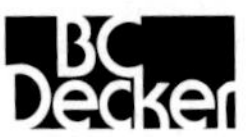

07 08 09/WPC/9 8 7 6 5 4 3 2 1

ISBN 978-1-55009-383-4
Printed in the United States of America by Walsworth Publishing Company

Sales and Distribution

United States
BC Decker Inc
P.O. Box 785
Lewiston, NY 14092-0785
Tel: 905-522-7017; 800-568-7281
Fax: 905-522-7839; 888-311-4987
E-mail: info@bcdecker.com
www.bcdecker.com

Canada
BC Decker Inc
50 King St. E.
P.O. Box 620, LCD 1
Hamilton, Ontario L8N 3K7
Tel: 905-522-7017; 800-568-7281
Fax: 905-522-7839; 888-311-4987
E-mail: info@bcdecker.com
www.bcdecker.com

Foreign Rights
John Scott & Company
International Publishers' Agency
P.O. Box 878
Kimberton, PA 19442
Tel: 610-827-1640
Fax: 610-827-1671
E-mail: jsco@voicenet.com

Japan
Igaku-Shoin Ltd.
Foreign Publications Department
3-24-17 Hongo
Bunkyo-ku, Tokyo, Japan 113-8719
Tel: 3 3817 5680
Fax: 3 3815 6776
E-mail: fd@igaku-shoin.co.jp

UK, Europe, Scandinavia,
Middle East
Elsevier Science
UK, Europe, Scandinavia,
Middle East, Africa
Elsevier Ltd.
Books Customer Services
Linacre House
Jordan Hill
Oxford
OX2 8DP, UK
Tel: 44 (0) 1865 474 010
Fax: 44 (0) 1865 474 011
E-mail: eurobkinfo@elsevier.com

Singapore, Malaysia, Thailand,
Philippines, Indonesia, Vietnam,
Pacific Rim, Korea
Elsevier Science Asia
583 Orchard Road
#09/01, Forum
Singapore 238884
Tel: 65-737-3593
Fax: 65-753-2145

Australia, New Zealand
Elsevier Science Australia
Customer Service Department
Locked Bag 16
St. Peters, New South Wales 2044
Australia
Tel: 61 02-9517-8999
Fax: 61 02-9517-2249
E-mail: customerserviceau@
elsevier.com
www.elsevier.com.au

Mexico and Central America
ETM SA de CV
Calle de Tula 59
Colonia Condesa
06140 Mexico DF, Mexico
Tel: 52-5-5553-6657
Fax: 52-5-5211-8468
E-mail: editoresdetextosmex@
prodigy.net.mx

Brazil
Tecmedd Importadora E
Distribuidora De Livros Ltda.
Avenida Maurílio Biagi, 2850
City Ribeirão, Ribeirão Preto –
SP – Brasil
CEP: 14021-000
Tel: 0800 992236
Fax: (16) 3993-9000
E-mail: tecmedd@tecmedd.com.br

India, Bangladesh, Pakistan,
Sri Lanka
Elsevier Health Sciences Division
Customer Service Department
17A/1, Main Ring Road
Lajpat Nagar IV
New Delhi – 110024, India
Tel: 91 11 2644 7160-64
Fax: 91 11 2644 7156
E-mail: esindia@vsnl.net

Dedication

Whoever would be a teacher...
let him begin by teaching himself...
and let him teach by example.
Kahil Gibran

Such a book would not be possible would not it have been for those who have taught me. Professionally, to Dr. George Adams and Dr. Sylvan Stool, sorely missed but never forgotten; the Faculty at the University of Minnesota; my teachers and current colleagues at the University of Pittsburgh and Children's Hospital of Pittsburgh, and most of all, the children and their families who extend the privilege of their care to me and in so doing teach me new things every day. Also to those who taught me everything else – Michael and Julie –Joseph, Sadie, Emad, and Philomena in my heart now and forever.

Joseph E. Dohar, MD, MS, FACS, FAAP

Preface

Nearly 100 years ago, Dr. R. F. Harrell of Alexandria wrote that "*otitis externa acuta*" is caused by:

> *Catching cold, especially being exposed to strong draughts of damp air…*
> — Dr. R. F. Harrell,
> The New Orleans Medical and Surgical Journal, 1908

What a difference a century makes! Admittedly, we have learned a great deal about the etiology, treatment, and prevention of otitis externa since the time of this assertion. Thousands of studies and articles have been published since Dr. Harrell's article, but the results of these studies and articles are often conflicting, difficult to interpret, and impractical for practicing physicians to implement. Complicating matters further are guidelines that promote themselves as independent but are funded by sources not free from conflict of interest. Even worse, some "guidelines" threaten to serve as a springboard for performance measures, a relatively new approach to attempt to determine whether consistent high-quality medical care is provided across health care systems. It would be a text unto itself to discuss the perils and pitfalls of both of these constructs, but they are nonetheless realities in our current medical climate.

Why this book on otitis externa? In my academic career, I have focused much of my attention on the study of the draining ear. I have been privileged to educate thousands of health care providers and have been asked the questions that commonly arise in a primary care setting. While the answers to some have been published long ago, others rely on information newly available.

To try to address these needs in a format that is convenient, practical, and educational, *PDQ Otitis Externa* was born. To quote Dr. Harrell again:

> *In my selection of a subject for this occasion, I have been actuated largely by a desire to present something that would be of interest to the general practitioner. As these cases most always fall into the hands of the general practitioner first, I have felt that a discussion of some of the practical points connected with the disease could hardly fail to elicit the general interest of this body.*

Nearly 100 years later, I find that some things are not so different and I could not agree more!

Contents

Definition and Etiology

The affection presents itself in two forms, namely: Circumscribed and diffuse inflammation of the canal.

— Dr. R. F. Harrell,
The New Orleans Medical and Surgical Journal, 1908

DEFINITION

Otitis externa (OE) is a broad term that includes inflammation, often due to infection, of the external auditory canal (EAC). It literally refers to any inflammatory process of the EAC. OE encompasses a wide range of diseases, and the most frequent type of OE is a common inflammatory infection of the EAC that can spread to the pinna and even the temporal bone if not treated correctly. Dermal swelling, epidermal thickness, and vascular dilation characterize the inflammation. It can range from a mild inflammation to necrotizing OE, a potentially life-threatening disease in older adults.

Inflammation vs. Infection

It is critical to emphasize at the outset of this text that *inflammation*, not infection or other factors, is pathognomonic of OE. This is important since all too often the emphasis for this disease is on eradication of infectious organisms. Although it is true that most cases of OE are due to bacterial infections that must be eradicated, it is the inflammation that is responsible for the signs and symptoms, for the complications, and for most of the treatment failures. Inflammation is the fundamental element of diagnosis and crucial to consider when making treatment decisions.

> **PDQ fact:** *Although it is true that most cases of otitis externa are due to bacterial infections that must be eradicated, it is the inflammation that is responsible for the signs and symptoms, for the complications, and for most of the treatment failures.*

Classification

OE can be subdivided into:

- Acute
- Recurrent-acute
- Chronic

More commonly, and of greater practical significance, OE can also be characterized as follows:

- Swimmer's ear — formally called *acute diffuse bacterial otitis externa* (and often shortened to *acute otitis externa*); it affects the entire ear canal
- *Furuncle* — an outer ear infection where only a part of the ear canal is swollen
- *Chronic eczematous otitis externa* — the outer ear is inflamed but not because of an infection; similar to eczema of the scalp
- Fungal – also known as *otomycosis*
- *Viral otitis externa* – also known as *herpes zoster oticus*
- *Necrotizing otitis externa* – also known as *skull base osteomyelitis*; referred to in the past as *"malignant" otitis externa*

Acute Inflammatory Phase

The acute exudative inflammatory phase of a nonspecific inflammation is marked by swelling and the presence of fetid debris that can develop into a nidus for Gram-negative bacteria and anaerobes. Swelling of the postauricular lymph nodes and postauricular extension of the erythema and edema might also occur and is sometimes referred to as "pseudomastoiditis." This clinical presentation is referred to as "pseudomastoiditis" because the condition is often misdiagnosed as *mastoiditis*. True mastoiditis does not develop, but the soft tissue overlying the postauricular region can be significantly inflamed and painful. There is distinct loss of the postauricular skin crease. In such cases it is critical to consider definitive imaging studies (i.e., CT scan) if physical examination and history alone cannot make the distinction. To complicate matters further, "pseudomastoiditis" can present concomitant with and as a complication of otitis media. These variable presentations will be described more fully in the case reports at the end of this book.

Chronic Inflammatory Phase

The acute phase is followed by the chronic inflammatory phase, which is characterized by atrophic epithelium, intense pruritus, and a superinfection accompanied by acute *dermatitis*. Conversely, rather than atrophic changes in the skin, the skin may become thickened. In extreme cases, chronic *osteitis* of the bone of the EAC may result in *stenosis* of the ear canal (Figure 1-1). *Perichondritis* also occurs in some cases. Clinicians should try to prevent these latter complications. Keys to such prevention are early diagnosis and aggressive treatment of acute OE so that it does not progress to chronic OE or extend to periauricular tissues such as the cartilaginous framework of the auricle.

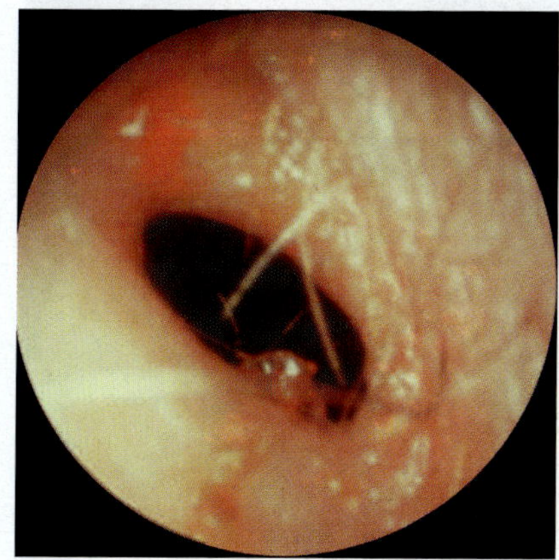

Figure 1-1. External auditory canal stenosis. Stenosis of the ear canal can result from chronic osteitis of the bone of the external auditory canal.

Pathophysiology Influences Treatment Strategies

Most types of OE have both acute and chronic forms that may differ pathophysiologically and thus require different treatment strategies. *Acute diffuse bacterial OE* is a bacterial infection and the most common type of OE in the United States (Figure 1-2). It generally responds well to treatment. On the other hand, *chronic bacterial OE* does not respond quickly to antibiotic therapy (Figure 1-3). In many cases, it does not respond at all to antibiotics. This may be true even where culture is obtained and the pathogens that are isolated are other than what would be expected to comprise the normal flora of the healthy EAC.

Incidence

In the United States, the incidence of acute OE is cited as affecting 4/1,000/year, of which 1% (4/100,000) progresses to become chronic. This equates to over

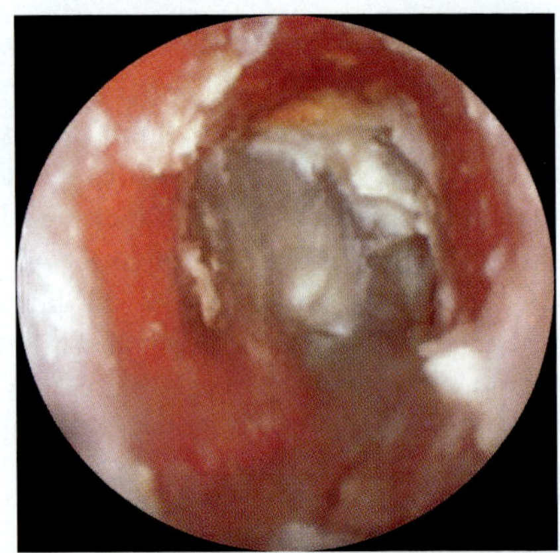

Figure 1-2. Acute diffuse bacterial otitis externa. The most common type of otitis externa in the U.S., it is often characterized by a copious, creamy exudate that fills the medial canal. The underlying skin is erythematous and edematous.

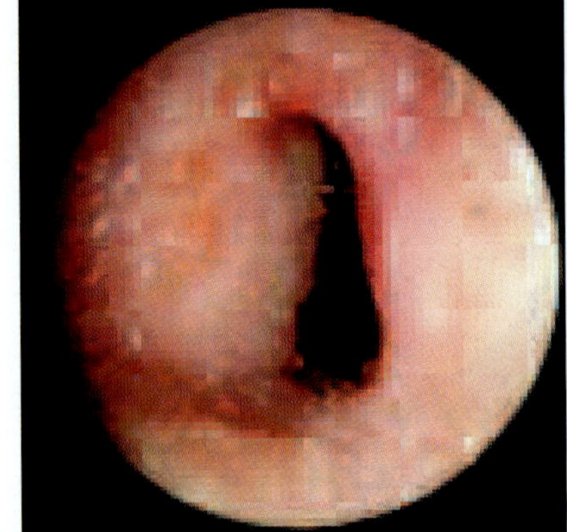

Figure 1-3. Chronic bacterial otitis externa. In many cases, chronic bacterial otitis externa does not respond at all to antibiotics.

five million cases a year treated by American primary care physicians. Acute diffuse bacterial OE is five times more common in swimmers than in non-swimmers and rarely affects both ears (an incidence of 20%).

PDQ fact: *American primary care physicians treat 5 million cases of acute otitis externa a year.*

Otitis Externa or Otitis Media?

Often, clinicians struggle with the diagnostic challenge of distinguishing the various types of OE not only from one another but also from the common types of otitis media. A summary of the key clinical distinctive features are listed below. Additional detail is provided in Chapter 3.

Otitis Externa

- **Acute bacterial** — scanty white mucoid discharge (occasionally thick)
- **Chronic bacterial** — can be bloody; granulation tissue is often present
- **Fungal** — white to off-white discharge, but may be black, gray, bluish-green, or yellow; black or white conidiophores on white hyphae are associated with *Aspergillus*

Otitis Media (with Perforated Tympanic Membrane)

- **Acute** – purulent white to yellow mucus with deep pain
- **Serous** – clear mucus, especially in the presence of allergies
- **Chronic** – intermittent purulent mucus without pain
- **Cerebrospinal fluid leak** – clear, thin, and watery discharge
- **Trauma** – bloody mucus
- **Osteomyelitis** – granulation tissue and discharge; odor-imaging studies may be needed

ETIOLOGY

The cause of OE is usually infectious although non-infectious and dermatological processes should not be forgotten. Before World War II, interest in studying the etiology of this disease was minimal and OE was believed to be caused by fungal infection. However, during the war, OE entered the medical spotlight because it was prevalent among American troops in the South Pacific. This disease became the second most common reason for lost duty among troops stationed in Guam. Microbiologic studies initiated during World War II established that OE is primarily bacterial in origin rather than fungal, which has been confirmed by subsequent studies.

Currently, OE occurs more frequently during the "swimming season," i.e., the summer months.

Common Bacterial Pathogens

Of the infectious causes, 80% are bacterial (Figure 1-4). The most common bacterial pathogens are:

- *Pseudomonas aeruginosa* (most common)
- *Staphylococcus aureus* and
- Other Gram-negative organisms such as Enterococcus species and *Proteus mirabilis*

These pathogens are in striking contrast to those that constitute the flora of the normal healthy external ear canal of which 96% are Gram-positive organisms (*Staphylococcus epidermidis*, Coryneforms, and streptococci-like species).

A recent study reported on microbiology specimens collected from 2,039 subjects (2,240 diseased ears) by 101 investigators throughout the United States (Figure 1-5). A total of 2,838 bacteria, 32 yeasts, and 17 molds were recovered from 2,048 ears clinically diagnosed as acute OE. Of the 202 bacterial species recovered, the species most frequently isolated were:

- *P. aeruginosa* (38%)
- *S. epidermidis* (9.1%)
- *S. aureus* (7.8%)
- *Microbacterium otitidis* (6.6%)
- *Microbacterium alconae* (2.9%)
- *Staphylococcus caprae* (2.6%)
- *Staphylococcus auricularis* (2.0%)
- *Enterococcus faecalis* (1.9%)
- *Enterobacter cloacae* (1.6%)
- *Staphylococcus capitis* subsp. Ureolyticus (1.4%) and
- *Staphylococcus haemolyticus* (1.3%)

It is important to understand what are considered normal flora in the EAC since this serves as a basis for understanding what bacteria are pathogenic. There is debate over whether or not certain bacteria such as *S. aureus* are pathogenic. If those bacteria are clearly different than those comprising normal flora, they can be considered potential pathogens.

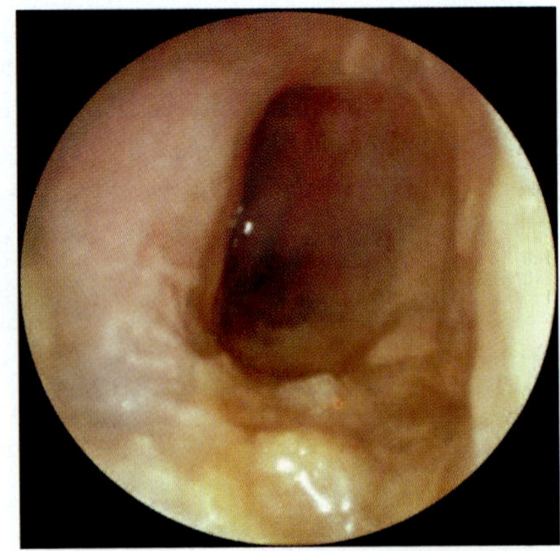

Figure 1-4. Acute bacterial otitis externa. In this case, purulent debris partially occludes the external canal. The yellow-green color leads one to suspect *P. aeruginosa*, the most common bacterial pathogen.

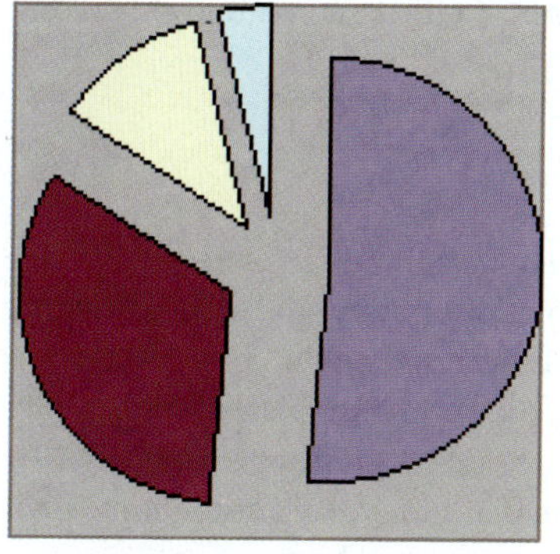

Figure 1-5. Bacterial pathogens. A recent study reported on microbiology specimens collected from 2,039 subjects (2,240 diseased ears) by 101 investigators. The following represents the species most frequently isolated from the 202 bacterial species recovered.

Susceptibility Profiles

Susceptibility profiles of *S. epidermidis* isolates revealed the greatest frequency of high-level resistance to selected antibiotics (>/=8 microg/mL):

- Neomycin-resistant (23%)
- Oxacillin-resistant (11%) and
- Ofloxacin-resistant (12%)

Susceptibility profiles of *S. aureus* isolates revealed a lower frequency of high-level resistance:

- Neomycin-resistant (6.3%)
- Oxacillin-resistant (2.7%) and
- Ofloxacin-resistant (4.5%)

P. aeruginosa with high-level resistance to quinolones ($\geq$ 128 mcg/mL for ofloxacin) was recovered from only one subject. Likewise, resistance of *P. aeruginosa* to aminoglycosides was rare. Twenty isolates had neomycin MICs $\geq$ 64 mcg/mL and 10 isolates had gentamicin MICs $\geq$ 16 mcg/mL. The coryneform isolates identified as *M. otitidis* had an intrinsic lack of susceptibility to quinolones (ofloxacin MICs $\geq$16 mcg/mL) and aminoglycosides (tobramycin MICs $\geq$ 32 mcg/mL and gentamicin MICs $\geq$ 8 mcg/mL).

Emergent Causes

As taxonomy in microbiology continues to change, advance, and evolve and as identification methodologies become more specific and precise, new organisms not traditionally listed as causes of OE are emerging. One recent example is *Malassezia sympodialis*.

Fungi

Fungi such as *Candida albicans* and *Aspergillus fumigatus*, when found, are generally considered pathogens and not saprophytes given their distinct absence from healthy ear canals. Much has been said to the contrary and it is critical to keep this in mind as few of the common ototopical therapies have anti-fungal spectrums of activity. Fungi are said to cause approximately 10% of cases of acute OE. Experience suggests that fungi play a more important role in chronic infections and immunocompromised hosts.

Though not confirmed, there is increasing concern that prolonged treatment with certain broad-spectrum ototopical antibiotics such as those from the quinolone class may also be a risk factor for development of fungal OE. It is clear that, not unlike the spectrum of fungal disease in the paranasal sinuses, fungi in the ear can behave similarly. Specifically, fungi may be present as saprophytes or may cause invasive non-fulminant and invasive fulminant disease. Lastly, there is increasing evidence that *allergic fungal otitis* is a distinct and real entity conferring yet another potential role for fungi in OE.

Viruses

Viruses may also cause acute OE. The most important cause of viral acute otitis media is *herpes zoster oticus*, referred to as Ramsay-Hunt syndrome when

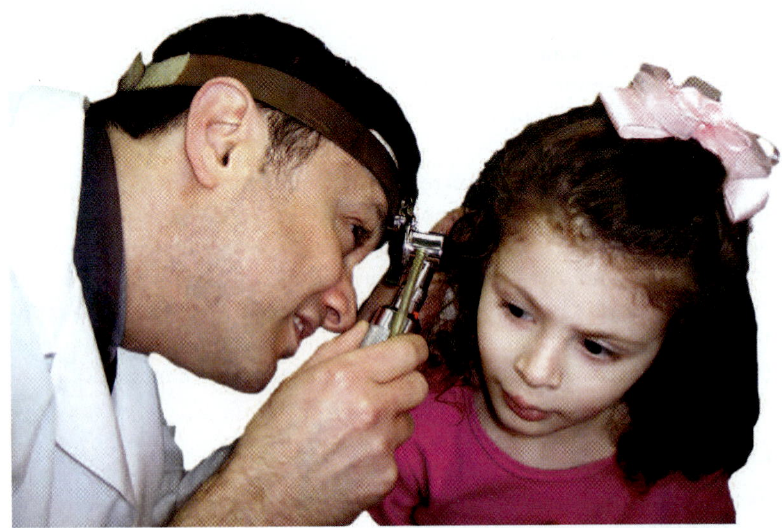

facial paralysis, hearing loss, and vertigo result. Vesicular eruptions delineate a viral etiology from a bacterial or fungal one. Another viral form of acute OE is *otitis externa hemorrhagica* (*bullous myringitis*). Physical signs of hemorrhagic bulla on the tympanic membrane are pathognomonic.

To Culture or Not To Culture?

There is debate regarding the value of culture in OE. A recent study concluded that "the result of the swab from the diseased ear did not change management in 96% of patients reviewed." This is likely true in most instances. Cultures are important in:

- Refractory cases
- Recurrent cases
- Cases where the disease extends beyond the confines of the EAC and
- Cases where suppurative complications have occurred
- Cases where certain co-morbid factors (ie. diabetes or immunocompromise) increase the likelihood of the need for systemic antibiotics

Cultures may be of value in diagnosis and in treatment, especially where adjunctive systemic treatment may be indicated. More information regarding the role of culture in diagnosis and treatment is in Chapter 4.

SUMMARY

OE is a broad term that includes inflammation, often due to infection, of the EAC. OE encompasses a wide range of diseases ranging from a furuncle on part of the ear canal to the potential deadly skull base osteomyelitis. Physicians treat more than 5 million cases a year, with children as predominant sufferers. Of the infectious causes of OE, 80% are bacterial, with *P. aeruginosa* as the most comment bacterial pathogen.

FLASHBACK

One hundred years ago, the average life expectancy in the United States was 47 years, only 14% of U.S. homes had bathtubs, and only 8% had telephones.

Anatomy, Physiology, and Pathogenesis

Otorrhea dependent on disease of the deeper structures which contain cocco-bacteria…the presence of fungi growing in the canal…more frequently the cause of the diffuse…form of the disease. The use of vegetable oils, such as castor and sweet oil, favors the development of these fungi…Chronic eczema of the canal, in those employed in slaughter-pens, will often…bring on the disease.

—Dr. R. F. Harrell,
The New Orleans Medical and Surgical Journal, 1908

ANATOMY AND PHYSIOLOGY

To understand the pathophysiology by which the previously described pathogens cause acute OE, one must understand the normal anatomy and physiology of the EAC.

Structure Influences Susceptibility to Disease

The unique structure of the EAC contributes to the development of OE. It is unique in that it is the only skin-lined cul-de-sac in the body. Its lateral one-third is cartilaginous; the medial two-thirds is bony (Figure 2-1). This is the opposite of the composition of the eustachian tube. The skin overlying the bony canal is thin and quite susceptible to trauma. It is exquisitely susceptible to pain. The EAC is warm, similar to core body temperature, making it one accepted site for measurement of this vital sign. It may also be humid. Exfoliated skin provides an ideal growth medium for bacteria and fungi.

The skin of the EAC is unique in that it is continually migrating laterally from the tympanic membrane outward, carrying debris with it. The exit of

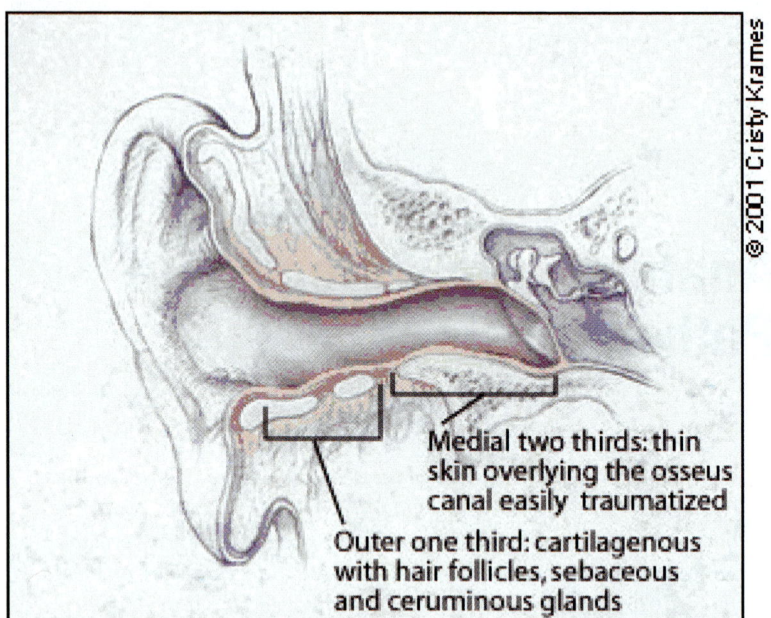

Figure 2-1. Anatomy of the external auditory canal. The unique structure of the external auditory canal contributes to the development of otitis externa. Accessed at: http://www.aafp.org/afp/20010301927-f1.jpg

debris, secretions, and foreign bodies is impeded by a curve at the junction of the cartilage and bone.

Role of Cerumen

Lipid-rich cerumen is protective in that it is acidic (pH 6.1-6.4) and hydrophobic (prevents water from penetrating to the skin and causing maceration). Cerumen is produced by the dermal adnexal structures called pilosebaceous glands. In addition, it contains lysozymes that inhibit bacterial growth. The normal EAC should be self-cleaning. When it is not, there are a variety of ways of removing cerumen including irrigation, suction, mechanical removal, and cerumenolytics. However, too much or too little cerumen predisposes to acute OE. Too little cerumen can predispose the ear canal to infection, but cerumen that is excessive or too viscous can lead to obstruction, retention of water and debris, and infection.

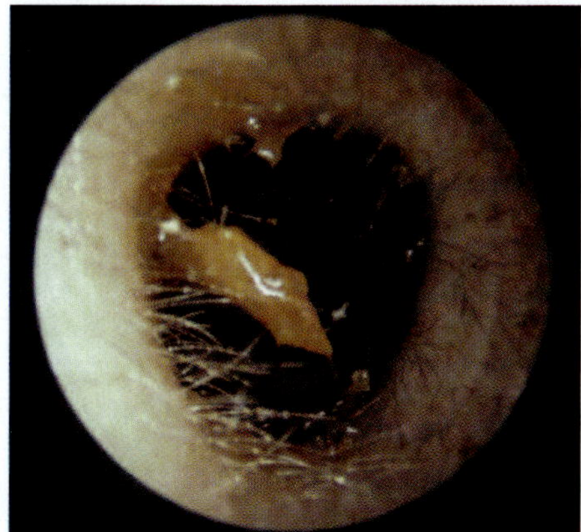

Figure 2-2. Normal cerumen. The ceruminous glands are modified sweat glands located in the outer cartilaginous canal. These glands produce a clear, colorless secretion that is properly called "cerumen." In most individuals, the secretions of the ceruminous glands and the outwardly migrating keratin squames continue to migrate laterally and are spontaneously discharged from the external canal by the normal process of migration.

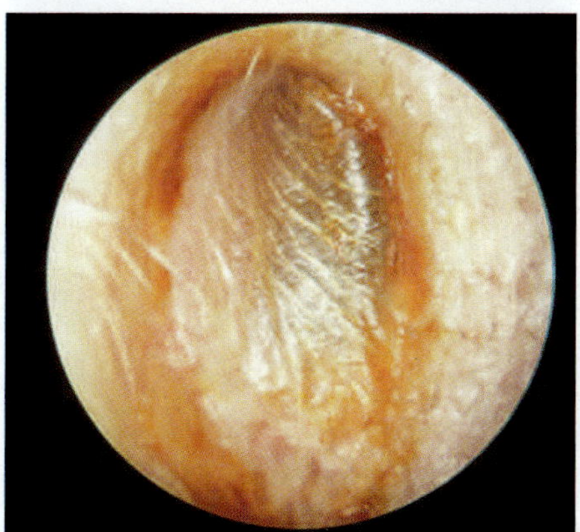

Figure 2-3. Veil of cerumen. In some individuals, a thin "veil" of cerumen will be seen draped across the lumen of the EAC. These patients will complain of hearing loss if the veil completely seals off the canal. Such a veil is usually the result of the insertion of a cotton-tipped applicator that has elevated and rotated the superficial layer of outwardly migrating keratin.

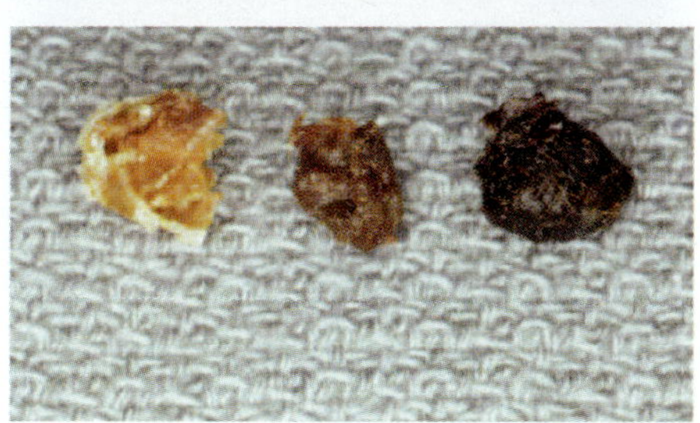

Figure 2-4. The colors of cerumen. Normal cerumen varies in color from a light golden yellow through brown to black.

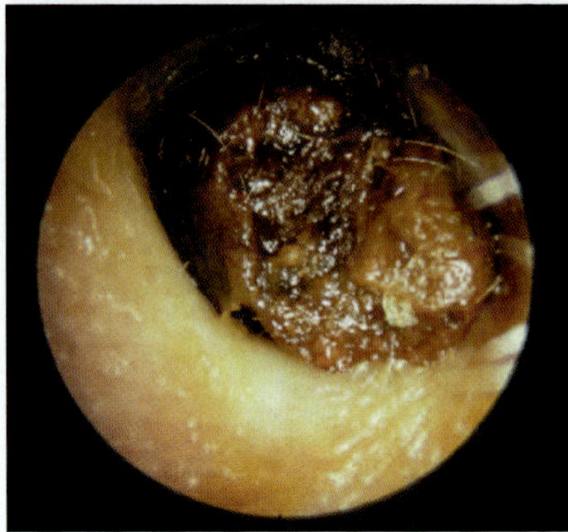

Figure 2-5. Cerumen accumulation. The ear canal is often occluded by cerumen (earwax), which must be removed if the entire tympanic membrane is to be seen and a proper otoscopic examination accomplished. Although cerumen is normally removed from the external canal by the process of epithelial migration, in some patients, there is a failure of migration, which results in cerumen accumulation within the canal.

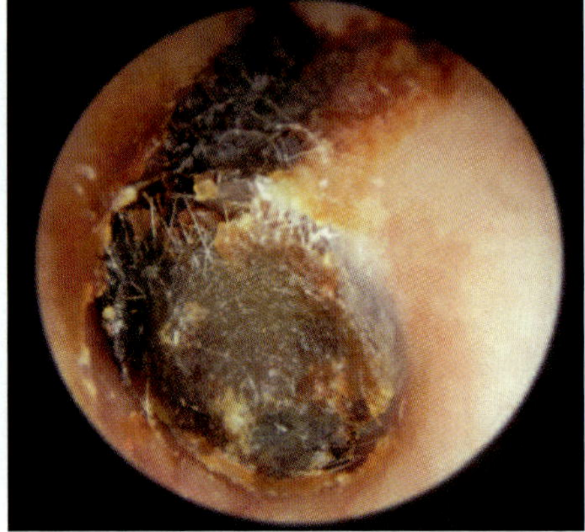

Figure 2-6. Cotton swab abuse. Individuals who frequently use cotton swabs to clean their ears often push their cerumen back into the deep meatus until it lies directly against the tympanic membrane. In these circumstances, loosening of the cerumen with an effective cerumenolytic prior to syringing is advisable.

PATHOGENESIS

The pathogenesis of nonspecific inflammation involves a maceration of the meatal skin as a result of mechanical or chemical damage. The consequences include a reduction in skin elasticity, atrophy and/or decreased output of the ceruminous and sebaceous glands, the loss of protective films and secretions, and a chemical imbalance (i.e., a pH level >6).

Primary Predisposing Factor

Many do not realize that acute OE is most often initiated by the alteration of the EAC pH and moisture. The high pH level in patients with nonspecific inflammation support the growth of bacteria and fungi. It is, therefore, most commonly seen during the hot and humid summer months.

It has mistakenly been thought that water exposure leads to acute OE due to bacterial contamination of the water that then infects the EAC upon entry. This is now known to be untrue. The actual mechanism by which water entry leads to acute OE is in altering the physiologic pH of the EAC toward increased alkalinity. Thus it is factors that raise the pH, such as water, humidity, or removal of cerumen, that predispose the EAC to infection.

PDQ fact: *It is factors that raise the pH, such as water, humidity, or removal of cerumen, that predispose the external auditory canal to infection.*

Secondary Predisposing Factors

Other predisposing factors may serve to breach the defenses of the lining epithelium and enable organisms to gain a foothold and cause infection. The following is a list of secondary factors:

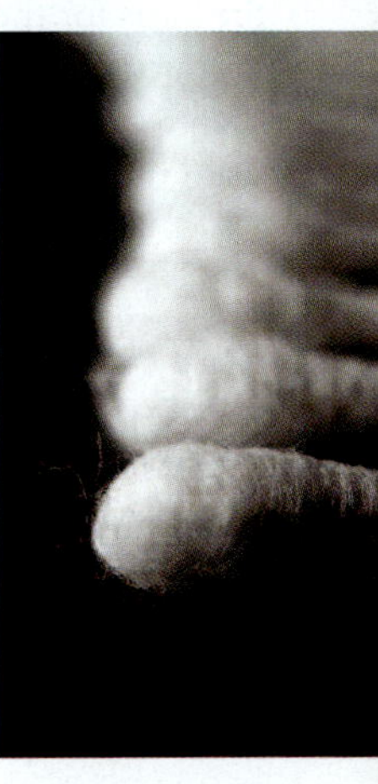

- Anatomy – a narrow canal, excessive wax production
- Moisture – swimming, perspiration, high humidity
- High environmental temperatures
- Mechanical removal of cerumen
- Trauma – e.g., cotton-buds, fingernails, hearing aids, ear plugs, hair grips, paper clips etc.
- Hair – some hair helps obviate entry of foreign bodies into the EAC, but the presence of thicker hair (common in older men) can be an impediment to EAC self-cleaning
- Chronic dermatological disease – e.g., eczema, psoriasis, seborrheic dermatitis, acne
- Immunocompromised host — e.g., diabetic
- Prior radiotherapy
- Contaminated water (possibly)

Hospitalization as a Predisposing Factor

Although not traditionally listed as a risk factor, patients who stayed more than 15 days in an intensive care unit were at increased risk of developing acute OE. Also, during critical illness, major alterations in cellular and humoral functions of the body are known to occur. Secretion of cytokines, hormones, and catecholamines may be disturbed. Finally, critically ill patients are usually immobile and must be washed in bed. During washing procedures, entrance of water into the EAC is usually inevitable and may be an important predisposing factor in the development of OE. Cleaning the EAC with a cotton-tipped applicator may be another cause of OE in intensive care units.

Medication as a Predisposing Factor

Widely used agents such as dopamine, epinephrine, or norepinephrine may alter the immune response of the body. If these alterations are prolonged and intense, the risk of infection will increase. Furthermore, overprescribing of antibiotics either for a prophylaxis or a treatment of a known infection alters the normal ecological flora of patients. The normal flora of the EAC is no exception.

SUMMARY

When defenses fail or when the epithelium of the EAC is damaged, OE results. There are many precipitants of this infection, but the most common is excessive moisture that elevates the pH and removes the cerumen. Once the protective cerumen is removed, keratin debris absorbs the water, creating a nourishing medium that supports bacterial growth. These concepts serve as the basis for the predisposition to recurrent OE in patients whose cerumen production is down-regulated. Prophylactic strategies are indicated to prevent such recurrences while attempting to restore normal physiologic homeostasis to the EAC, which is far more delicate and balanced than many realize.

> **FLASHBACK**
> One hundred years ago, Alabama, Mississippi, Iowa, and Tennessee were each more populated than California.

Diagnosis

3

I remember being called a few years ago to consult with a very intelligent general practitioner in a case of this kind, where he had suspected mastoid involvement. On careful examination, it was found that the whole trouble came from a case of inflammation of the external auditory canal.

—Dr. R. F. Harrell,
The New Orleans Medical and Surgical Journal, 1908

A recent set of guidelines has been published that define the elements of diagnosis of OE as follows:

- Rapid onset (within 48 hours) in the past 3 weeks
- *Symptoms* of ear canal inflammation
  - Otalgia (often severe)
  - Itching
  - Fullness
  - ± hearing loss or jaw pain
- *Signs* of ear canal inflammation
  - Tragal tenderness and/or
  - Pinna tenderness
  - Diffuse EAC edema, erythema, or both
  - With or without otorrhea, regional lymphadenitis, tympanic membrane erythema, or cellulitis of the pinna and adjacent skin

MOST CHARACTERISTIC SYMPTOM AND SIGN

The most characteristic presenting *symptom* of OE is otalgia (ear discomfort) and the most characteristic *sign* is otorrhea (discharge in or coming from the EAC). It is important to keep in mind that although these symptoms and signs are also seen in otitis media with perforation or tympanostomy tube, they are inversely related to one another. In other words, in OE the otalgia is generally severe and the otorrhea scant. The opposite is true in otitis media in the face of a tympanic membrane perforation or tympanostomy tube.

The ear discomfort can range from pruritus to severe pain that is exacerbated by motion of the pinna or EAC, including chewing. If inflammation causes sufficient swelling to occlude the EAC, the patient may also complain of aural fullness and loss of hearing.

PDQ fact: *The most characteristic presenting symptom of otitis externa is otalgia and the most characteristic sign is otorrhea.*

The characteristics and qualities of otorrhea may be quite variable, especially in terms of odor, color, and consistency. Its characteristics often provide important clues to etiology. For example, scant white mucus that is generally quite viscous strongly suggests acute diffuse bacterial OE. Alternatively, bloody otorrhea with discharge suggests chronic OE and, if it fails to respond to appropriate therapy, must raise one's index of suspicion for benign tumors such as histiocytosis X, atypical pathogens such as mycobacterium, and malignancy. A fluffy discharge that is white, black, gray, blue-green, or yellow often suggests an otomycosis.

OTITIS EXTERNA OR OTITIS MEDIA?

The symptoms of acute OE are distinct and generally helpful in distinguishing it from acute otitis media, the key disease in the differential diagnosis. Although taken for granted, this distinction on physical examination alone is often not trivial. On the one hand, there may be so much swelling of the tissues related to the EAC that the tympanic membrane cannot be visualized. Even in cases where the tympanic membrane could and theoretically should be seen, the patient may have such severe pain that speculum insertion and auricular manipulation—normal steps in performing a pneumatic otoscopic examination—may not be tolerated or permitted. In cases of otitis media with otorrhea, copious amounts of pus in the EAC may preclude not only visualization of the tympanic membrane but also visualization of the EAC.

Also, both OE and otitis media can co-exist. If the tympanic membrane can be visualized and is red, pneumatic otoscopy or tympanometry may serve useful as diagnostic adjuncts in ascertaining whether associated otitis media is present. Special equipment such as an otomicroscope and suctioning apparatus may be needed. Further, adjunctive measures such as local and/or general anesthesia and imaging studies may also be needed. Even in the best of circumstances, misdiagnosis can and does occur.

AURAL TOILET INFLUENCES DIAGNOSIS

Otorrhea and other debris can occlude the ear canal and make it difficult to visualize the tympanic membrane and to exclude otitis media. It may also per-

Table 3-1.
Otitis media or otitis externa?

Symptom	Otitis externa	Otitis media
Outer ear redness	Often	Rare
Pain with manipulation of the ear	Intense	Rare
Discharge	Not very much	Considerable
Signs of respiratory infection (runny nose, congestion, sore throat, cough, fever, etc.)	Rare	Frequent

petuate a moist environment within the EAC which, in turn, interferes with topical treatment. It is imperative that good aural toilet be performed both for proper diagnosis and maximal treatment.

Mechanical Techniques

Inflammation renders the EAC even more vulnerable to trauma, and caution must be exercised when mechanical techniques such as those that make use of a cerumen curette are used in aural toilet (Figure 3-1). Aural toilet is best done by suctioning under direct visualization, using the open or operating

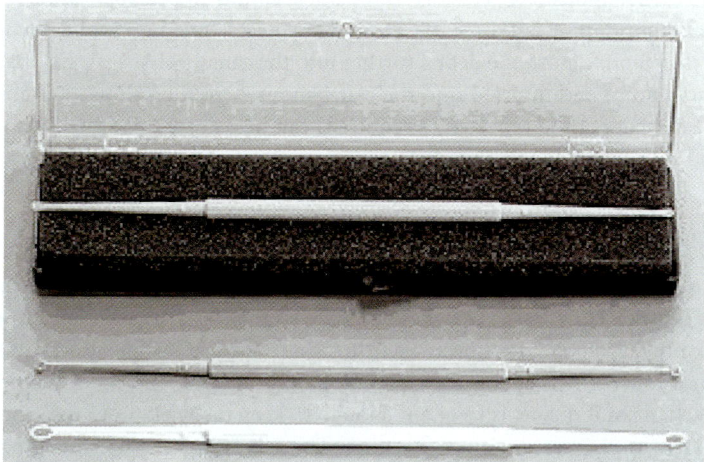

Figure 3-1. Cerumen curette. Accessed at: http://www.spectrumsurgical.com/catalog/instrument/curette.htm

otoscope head and a 5 or 7 French Frazier malleable suction tip attached to low suction (Figure 3-2). A microscope may also be useful in select circumstances. Unfortunately, such instrumentation is rarely available in a primary care setting and even if available, can be used only with sufficient training and experience.

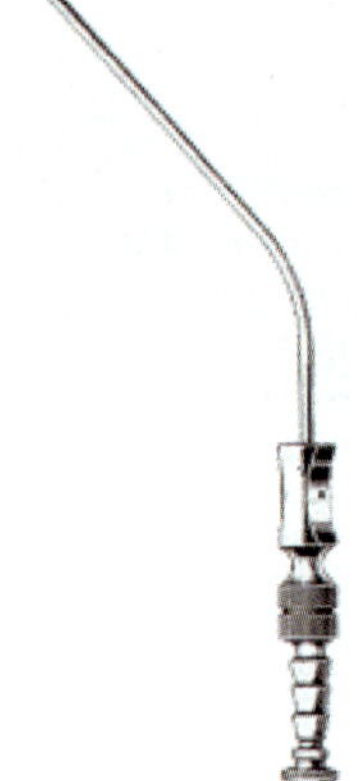

Figure 3-2. French Frazier suction tube. Accessed at: http://www.perfectra.com/allsuctiontube.htm

"Dry Mopping"

Studies show that "dry mopping" techniques are also effective in aural toilet. A cotton swab with the cotton fluffed out can be used to gently mop out thin secretions from the EAC, again under direct visualization. Commercially available Q-tips® rarely have value since they are designed to be larger than what reasonably can be advanced medially beyond the juncture of the bony and cartilaginous EAC. For this reason, most cotton-tipped applicators (other than for mopping out discharge around the meatal opening) are best avoided as they tend to push the debris further into the canal. "Tissue spears" twisted into a point and inserted into the canal about 2 cm then allowed to absorb the discharge (and repeated as required) can help absorb a serous discharge and thus facilitate more medial access prior to eardrop insertion.

Otowicks

If the EAC is so swollen that topical therapy cannot be effectively delivered, an otowick (or "wick") may be required (Figure 3-3). A wick serves to uniformly deliver the ototopical agent to the entire EAC while also providing aural toilet if it is changed frequently. Additionally, it allows for a delivery mechanism if dosing is frequent enough to keep the wick moist and continuously impregnated with medication. Though practices vary, changing the wick every 2 to 5 days with aural toilet is common practice. Smaller cotton-

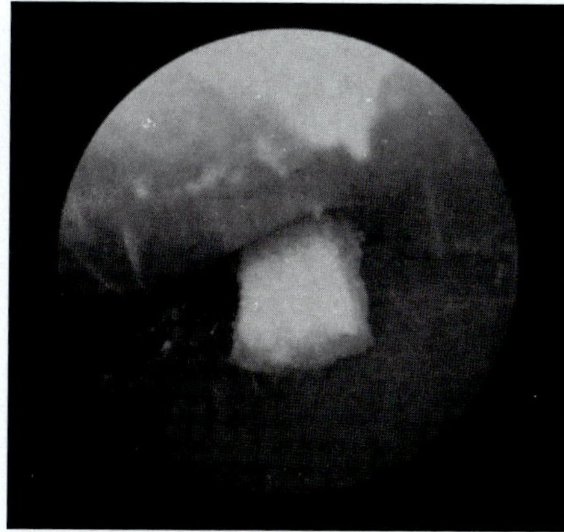

Figure 3-3. **An otowick**. A "wick" can uniformly deliver an ototopical agent to the entire external auditory canal and provide aural toilet if it is changed frequently.

tip applicators are available and are useful in cases where the dimensional anatomy of the EAC allow.

Antibiotic Drops

If the secretions are thick, crusted, or adherent, instillation of antibiotic drops may help solubilize some of the elements comprising it and thus expedite removal for aural toilet. Several other solvents have been advocated. It is important to keep in mind that inflamed skin is susceptible to irritation from many of these compounds and that, in the event that the tympanic membrane is not intact, ototoxicity may result.

Risk to Perforated Tympanic Membrane

Unless the tympanic membrane can be fully observed and is found to be intact, flushing of the ear canal should not be attempted. Such practice has met with catastrophic outcomes and poses substantial medical and legal risk. A small perforation is often missed, and a tympanic membrane already compromised by inflammation can be injured. Divers, surfers, and others who experience forceful compression of the tympanic membrane are particularly susceptible to perforations. "Syringing" the ear when the tympanic membrane is perforated can disrupt the ossicles and injure the cochlea and labyrinth, resulting in hearing loss, tinnitus, vertigo, and dizziness. Such trauma may necessitate surgery. In addition, flushing may cause further trauma to the ear canal or introduce EAC pathogens into the middle ear, thus advancing the infection to additional compartments not initially infected.

When External Auditory Canal Cleaning Isn't Possible

If the EAC cannot be easily cleaned because of swelling or pain, discharge and debris should be left in place and the patient should undergo frequent reevaluation until the secretions can be removed or have drained spontaneously.

CLINICAL DIFFERENTIAL DIAGNOSIS

Culture of the EAC may help to confirm the diagnosis though, practically speaking, is rarely obtained or needed. Since the primary sign of acute OE is otorrhea, it is important to know its differential diagnosis as this serves as the differential diagnosis for acute OE in general. Though not exhaustive and somewhat overlapping with classification, the most common conditions to consider are:

Infectious Causes
- Bacterial OE (most common)
- Fungal infection (otomycosis)
- Viral infection
  - Herpes simplex and herpes zoster (vesicles)

Noninfectious causes
- Allergic OE
  - Allergic contact dermatitis
  - Eczematous dermatitis (atopic dermatitis)
- Irritant contact dermatitis
- Psoriasis
- Seborrheic dermatitis
- Acne vulgaris
- Systemic lupus erythematosus

RULING OUT OTHER COMPLICATIONS

A thorough examination of the head and neck should always be performed to rule out other diagnoses and to look for possible complications of OE. The examination should include evaluation of the paranasal sinuses, nose, mastoids, temporomandibular joints, mouth, pharynx, and neck.

> **PDQ fact:** *A thorough examination of the head and neck should always be performed to rule out other diagnoses and to look for possible complications of otitis externa.*

SUMMARY

Although the most characteristic presenting *symptom* of OE is otalgia (ear discomfort) and the most characteristic *sign* is otorrhea (discharge in or coming from the EAC), practitioners now have an established set of guidelines that define the elements of diagnosis of OE. These diagnostic criteria are generally helpful in distinguishing OE from otitis media, which can be difficult even in a medical setting. Culture of the EAC may help to confirm the diagnosis though, practically speaking, is rarely obtained or needed.

Because otorrhea and other debris can make it difficult to visualize the tympanic membrane and even interfere with topical treatment, it is imperative that good aural toilet be performed. Several techniques exist, including mechanical techniques (using great care), "dry mopping," otowicks, and antibiotic drops if the tympanic membrane is intact. A thorough examination of the head and neck should always be performed to rule out other diagnoses and to look for possible complications of OE.

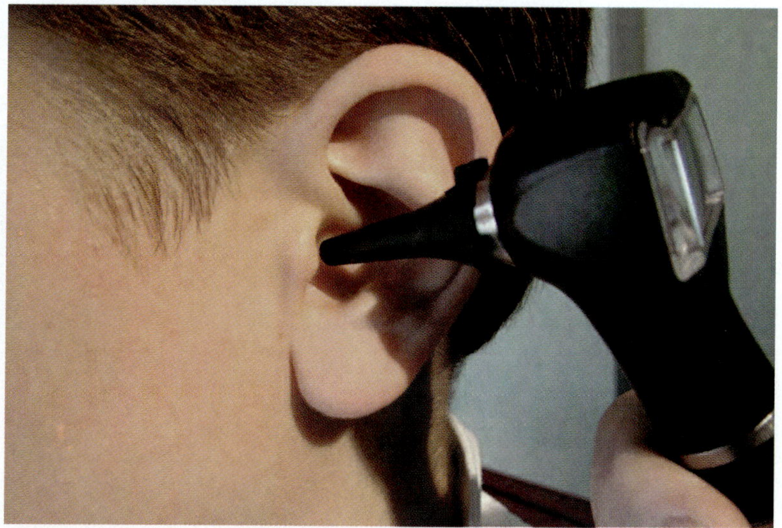

FLASHBACK

One hundred years ago, a 3-minute call from Denver to New York City cost $11. The maximum speed limit in most cities was 10 mph with only 8,000 cars in the United States, which were driven on only 144 miles of paved roads.

4

Management

The first efforts in the treatment of this affection are toward the relief of pain, and the absorption of the process before the stage of suppuration is reached.

—Dr. R. F. Harrell,
The New Orleans Medical and Surgical Journal, 1908

The treatment objectives for OE have remained consistent while treatment approaches have evolved. In this chapter, management of uncomplicated acute diffuse bacterial otitis externa is discussed. Chapter 6 describes the management of the other less common and advanced forms of OE.

GUIDELINES

A recent set of guidelines have been published that provide evidence-based recommendations for the management of diffuse acute OE (Table 4-1). This entity was defined in these guidelines as generalized inflammation of the EAC, which may also involve the pinna or tympanic membrane. The group made a *strong recommendation* that management should include an assessment of pain, and analgesic treatment should be recommended based on the severity of the pain.

Table 4-1.
Evidence-based guidelines for management of otitis externa

Rule out other causes for otalgia, otorrhea, inflammation
Identify factors that modify management: non-intact tympanic membrane, tympanostomy tube, diabetes, etc.
Use topical therapy first, based on efficacy, safety, compliance, cost
Use only non-ototoxic topical therapy if tubes/perforation are present
Teach patients/caregivers how to use topical agents, perform aural toilet
Reassess if no response to treatment after 48-72 hours
Use systemic antibiotics only when warranted

Recommendations were made that clinicians:

- Distinguish diffuse acute OE from other causes of otalgia, otorrhea, and inflammation of the ear canal
- Assess the patient with diffuse acute OE for factors that modify management such as a non-intact tympanic membrane, tympanostomy tube, diabetes mellitus, immunocompromise, and prior history of radiotherapy
- Use ototopical therapies as first-line, initial therapy for the treatment of diffuse, uncomplicated acute OE
- Reserve systemic therapy for extension beyond the EAC or for instances where specific host factors warrant systemic antibiotics

Additional Recommendations

- Choose topical agent based on efficacy, safety, compliance, and cost
- Treat patients with known tympanostomy tubes or perforations of the tympanic membrane with a non-ototoxic topical preparation (Ciprodex® Otic or Floxin® Otic)
- Instruct patients on proper delivery of the ototopical agent and aural toilet techniques
- Assess patients who fail to respond within 48-72 hours for proper diagnosis

GOALS OF THERAPY

The main goal of therapy is to eradicate the pathogens responsible for the infection while reducing ear pain. Earache is a common and significant symptom of OE, and its intensity is directly related to disease severity. Pain can be so severe that it results in the discontinuation of daily activities.

AURAL TOILET

As described in Chapter 3, it is imperative that good aural toilet be performed—not only for proper diagnosis but for maximal treatment, too. Most important is the removal of as much debris as possible. Chapter 3 described various methods, one of the best of which is suction (± microscopy), but "dry mopping" or gentle curettage provides an alternative.

Effective aural toilet improves patient outcomes (Table 4-2). In addition to the obvious benefit to diagnosis by allowing for direct inspection of the EAC, tympanic membrane, and middle ear, other therapeutic benefits to aural toilet exist, too. In order of importance, they are:

- **Drug delivery of ototopical therapies is markedly enhanced.** When the canal is quite swollen, an otowick helps facilitate drainage and enhance

Table 4-2.
Aural toilet improves patient outcomes

Drug delivery of ototopical therapies is enhanced
Bacterial colony counts are reduced
Normal physiologic homeostatic conditions are restored to the
  external auditory canal

delivery of ototopical medications. Even in the absence of swelling, oto-wicks markedly lengthen the resident time of medications in contact with the affected skin.

- **Bacterial colony counts are drastically reduced.** Aural toilet removes significant bacterial loads from the EAC, leaving less for the antibiotic and for the body's immune system and natural defenses to eradicate.
- **Normal physiologic homeostatic conditions are restored to the EAC.** This is a benefit sometimes not recognized. Normal homeostatic conditions include the restoration of pH, eradication of extracellular inflammatory mediators, and removal of potential survival substrates for infectious pathogens.

Aural Toilet in Special Populations

Aural toilet is especially important in children so that underlying causes of OE can be identified. This is particularly important when OE in young children (or those with psychiatric diagnoses) fail to resolve or recur. In such cases, foreign body must be aggressively sought.

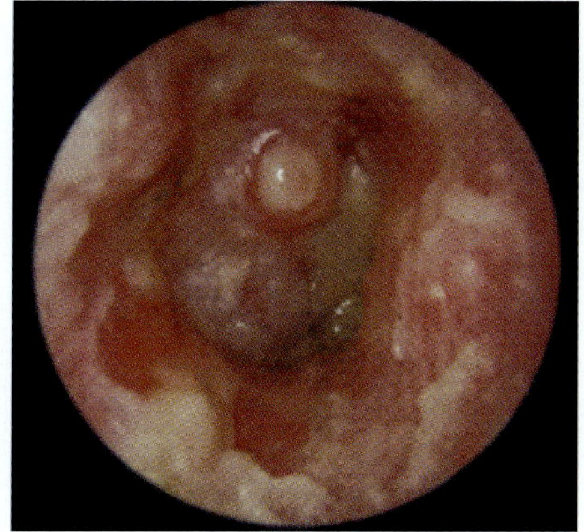

Severe acute aspergillus otitis externa. The underlying canal skin and tympanic membrane is often inflamed and ulcerated because of invasion by fungal mycelia. Refractory cases may require repeated aural toilet, with reapplication of the antifungal agent.

CULTURE

As discussed briefly in Chapter 1, culture and sensitivity are generally only indicated if the patient fails initial outpatient therapy with an appropriate medication (usually ototopical, as described later in this chapter). However, a culture should definitely be obtained if:

- The patient has co-morbid factors, including immunodeficiency that confers high risk for suppurative complications, local aggressive spread of infection, treatment failure, or recurrence
- Extension beyond the soft tissue of the EAC or
- Infection due to an atypical pathogen is suspected

During culture, the sample should be taken from the more medial aspect of the EAC to obviate sampling error. A wire/cotton swab should be used to reduce secondary bacterial contamination. Both bacterial and fungal stains and cultures should be obtained; obtain viral cultures in selected cases. Atypical pathogens and parasites are not routinely sought but may play a role in rare instances. Bacterial *in vitro* susceptibilities may not correlate with clinical outcomes since breakpoints are determined for systemic, not topical, administration; nevertheless, identifying the organism and distinguishing a fungal from a bacterial infection is of therapeutic significance.

> **PDQ fact:** *Topical therapy is the mainstay of management of otitis externa. At this time, the only FDA-approved combination topical agent that would be effective and safe if the integrity of the tympanic membrane is in question is ciprofloxacin/dexamethasone (Ciprodex® Otic).*

TOPICAL THERAPY

Topical therapy is the mainstay of management of OE. Though other therapies are described later in this chapter, this section will focus on the advantage of topical therapy over systemic therapy (in most cases) and the choice between combination formulations (combining multiple antibiotics, antibiotics and steroids, or both).

There are many advantages of using topical rather than systemic therapy (Table 4-3):

- Topical medications are delivered directly to the target organ
- Topical antibiotics are less likely to be a cause of bacterial resistance
- Topical antibiotics are less likely to be a cause of antibiotic resistance
- Topical therapy is generally used in relatively shorter treatment courses and
- Topical strategies benefit from fewer and more minor adverse events when compared to systemic antibiotics

Table 4-3.
Advantages of using topical therapy

Delivered directly to the target organ
Less likely to cause bacterial resistance
Less likely to cause antibiotic resistance
Shorter treatment courses
Fewer and more minor adverse events

Topical medications are delivered directly to the target organ

By bypassing the systemic circulation, pharmacokinetic variables such as solubility, intestinal absorption, and hepatic first pass effects, to name a few factors, do not affect ultimate tissue concentrations.

Topical antibiotics are less likely to be a cause of bacterial resistance

Short-term courses of treatment for superficial, community-acquired infections in otherwise healthy patients decrease the likelihood of resistance associated with topical antibiotic use. In general, these are the characteristics typically present when ototopical therapy is used to treat OE. Probably of greatest importance, however, is that ototopical medications can be readily delivered to the affected site in high concentrations. In fact, a likely explanation for reports citing the emergence of bacterial resistance to topical antibiotics is inadequate drug delivery. This has been reported in lower respiratory infections and in sinusitis where there is a substantial difference between the amount of topical drug administered and that which actually reaches the target organ. Generally speaking, this should not be the case in OE.

Topical antibiotics are less likely to be a cause of antibiotic resistance

The relative use of topical as compared to systemic antibiotics is so small that even if the two methods carried equal risk of contributing to antibiotic resistance, the topical contribution would be statistically insignificant. This point was corroborated by a study done in Pittsburgh. Two-hundred thirty-one consecutive children presenting to the outpatient otolaryngology clinic with draining ears from which *P. aeruginosa* was isolated were studied. Of these, 99.6% showed a sensitivity to polymyxin B, one of the active ingredients in Cortisporin® Otic,

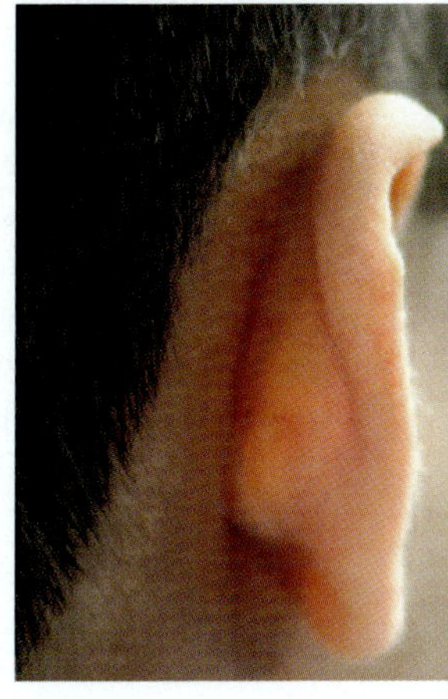

used very commonly in the community since the 1970s. Only one strain of *P. aeruginosa* proved resistant to polymyxin B. The authors concluded that despite widespread use of ototopical Cortisporin® Otic, which contains polymyxin B as one active ingredient in their community for nearly three decades, *P. aeruginosa*, known to be quite facile in developing resistance strategies, remained sensitive to it. One may argue that polymyxin B has distinct features rendering it less likely to become resistant. This failure to invoke resistance, however, has also been observed for topical skin antibiotics and topical eye drops as well with respect to antibiotics unlike polymyxin B that have been shown to be the target of resistance mechanisms quite readily. Crucial to this feature is that the concentrations of topical antibiotics exceeds the minimal inhibitory concentrations (MICs) at the site of infection to such a degree that eradication is more rapid and complete.

A recent report concluded that *P. aeruginosa*-resistance to ciprofloxacin (available in two ototopical formulations—Ciprodex® Otic and Cipro® HC Otic) increased in a select population of OE patients. The key here is that this is an agent in common use systemically and its systemic, not its ototopical, use is likely responsible for the emergence of increased resistance. When reports of resistance to a topical agent are made, a critical reviewer must carefully search for an explanation.

The two most commonly isolated pathogens from patients with OE, *P. aeruginosa* and *S. aureus*, are of major concern due to their propensity to develop resistance. In fact, methicillin-resistant *S. aureus* (MRSA) has now become not only a feared and challenging iatrogenic infection but also a frighteningly prevalent community-acquired infection amongst otherwise healthy patients. This, coupled with the relatively high prevalence of OE and the substantial public health concern that any bacterial resistance has become, strongly supports the development of strategies to minimize resistance in the future.

Topical therapy is generally used in relatively shorter treatment courses

Current trends are toward shorter treatment courses. The normal average is a week, and possibly less. Although pharmacokinetic and pharmacodynamic modeling specifically studying the use of topical antibiotics in ear disease has not been published, one can reasonably extrapolate from existing reports that the outcome of such studies are expected to be favorable. In addition, newer topical fluoroquinolones carry the added advantage of concentration-dependent killing. This would predictably have a clear advantage over time-dependent killers in topical delivery.

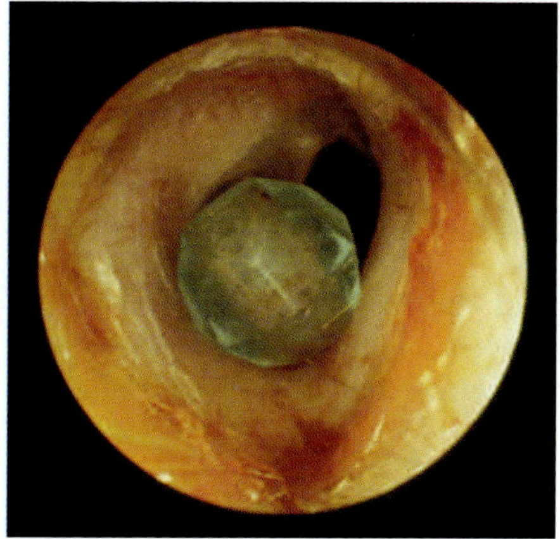

Foreign body: plastic bead. A wide variety of foreign bodies have been discovered in the external auditory canal. The symptoms will depend on the nature of the foreign body. Relatively inert materials may produce no symptoms and be discovered only inadvertently during a routine otoscopic examination, whereas organic material tends to cause a localized external otitis.

Topical strategies benefit from fewer and more minor adverse events when compared to systemic antibiotics

Newer Topical Agents

With the newer topical fluoroquinolone agents, only minor local irritative and allergic effects are common—a marked advantage. On the other hand, the product label of any systemic antibiotic will list such common side effects as diarrhea, nausea, rash, vomiting, abdominal pain, and headache, among others. Plus, far more severe side effects such as Stevens-Johnson syndrome, aplastic anemia, seizure, and anaphylaxis can occur as well. A recent trial comparing the efficacy and safety of topical ciprofloxacin/dexamethasone to amoxicillin/clavulanate found an incidence of 12.8% treatment-related side effects associated with the ototopical agent compared to 29.3% for the systemic agent. A similar study comparing topical ofloxacin to amoxicillin/clavulanate resulted in a similar reduced side-effect profile. The improved safety profile of topical over systemic antimicrobials is unequivocal.

Older Topical Agents

A higher incidence of adverse events has been reported for older ototopical agents such as Cortisporin® Otic. Most of these were local sensitivity responses and, by and large, were seen with neomycin-containing products. The major disadvantage of products containing neomycin is its propensity to lead to sensitization. This manifests as allergic inflammation, most often of the skin of the EAC and pinna. One study stated that "Because of the high risk of sensitization, topical preparations containing neomycin...should not be used routinely." Neomycin sensitization is likely underestimated. When used in the EAC, the package insert of Cortisporin® Otic, (PDR, 1995) states that the manifestation of sensitization to neomycin is usually a "low-grade reddening with swelling, dry scaling, and itching." It may manifest as "failure to heal." Given the experience in nasal allergy, it is known that epithelium responds to allergic triggers with edema and drainage. Clearly, in conditions such as OE, the inflammatory manifestations of allergy and infection are clinically similar, if not indistinguishable.

Similar problems have been noted with thimerosal, a common preservative found in older ototopical formulations. In a retrospective review of patch testing reactions from 587 adult patients, neomycin sulfate and thimerosal elicited a hypersensitivity reaction in 53% and 18% of the patients, respectively.

COMBINATION PRODUCTS

Multiple Antimicrobial Agents

Of current debate is the need for more than one antimicrobial agent in any single formulation. Cortisporin® Otic, Pediotic®, and Colymycin® are all examples of combination topical otic preparations that contain one or more antibiotics and an anti-inflammatory agent. These older combination drugs contain both neomycin and polymyxin B because neither drug alone is effective against *P. aeruginosa* and *S. aureus*.

However, the preference for minimizing the antibiotic components of therapy is driving physicians toward newer otic treatments, such as the fluoroquinolones, because physicians have been sensitized to the fact that multiple drugs increase the potential for adverse effects. The fluoroquinolones are preferred over combination drugs since their antimicrobial activities cover both pathogens when used as monotherapy.

Rationale for Combination Antibiotics

The rationale for the combination of antibiotics in some of these preparations is unclear. Polymyxin B sulfate (10,000 units per ml) represented in most topical ear preparations is effective against *P. aeruginosa* and other Gram-negative bacteria, including strains of *Escherichia*. Similarly, colistin sulfate (3 mg/mL) is effective against most Gram-negative organisms, notably *P. aeruginosa, Escherichia coli,* and *Klebsiella* species. Neomycin sulfate (3.3 mg/mL) is an aminoglycoside with primary effectiveness against many Gram-negative organisms and some activity against *S. aureus*. Surprisingly, from an anti-infective perspective, it is the activity against the Gram-positive staphylococci that led to the inclusion of neomycin—activity not generally emphasized for antibiotics belonging to the aminoglycoside class. The other

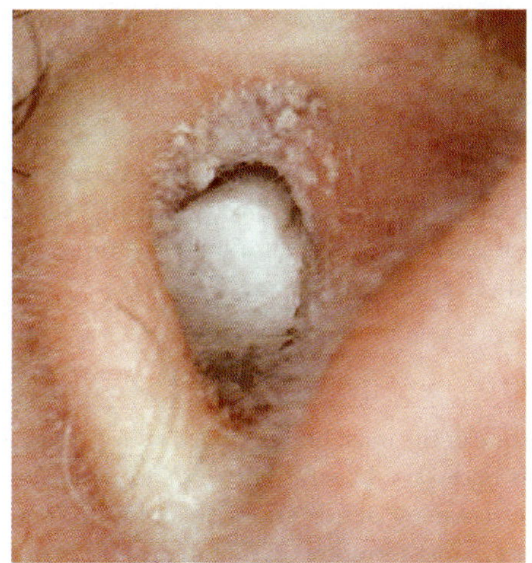

Pope Otowick inserted in an occluded ear canal (severe acute otitis externa). The wick should be replaced on a daily basis until the edema has subsided and the topical drops can be instilled directly into the canal. In the extremely severe case, the simultaneous administration of oral ciprofloxacin and a short course of high-dose prednisone may be beneficial. Appropriate analgesics and hypnotics are also indicated when acute otitis externa causes severe pain.

possible rationale for the inclusion of neomycin was to provide a second antibiotic with activity against Gram-negative bacteria such as the pseudomonas. It has been traditionally taught that "dual" antibiotic therapy is necessary when treating pseudomonas infections causing pneumonia or infection in immunocompromised patients. This premise has been based on the rationale that the synergy of two drugs with different modes of activity reduces the likelihood of treatment-induced resistance and more effectively eradicates the organism. This rationale also likely led to the development of combination ototopical agents containing an aminoglycoside (i.e., neomycin) and a member of the polymyxin class of antibiotics (i.e., polymyxin B sulfate).

Evidence Does Not Support Dual Therapy

Data on the treatment of aural pseudomonas infections have not supported the need for dual therapy systemically. A recent study from Pittsburgh revealed excellent *in vitro* susceptibility of aural isolates of *P. aeruginosa* to the semisynthetic penicillins. Single-agent intravenous therapy from this class of antibiotics has been the standard treatment for chronic suppurative otitis media due to *P. aeruginosa* in children, refractory to outpatient management, with excellent results.

The fluoroquinolones, as mentioned previously, achieve excellent coverage of both the Gram-positive and Gram-negative bacterial pathogens commonly recovered in OE and otitis media.

An *in vitro* analysis of antimicrobial activity against clinical isolates of *S. aureus* and *P. aeruginosa* indicated that ofloxacin and ciprofloxacin were more active against these pathogens than was neomycin. The MIC90 values of ofloxacin and ciprofloxacin, respectively, were 1.0 µg/mL and 2.0 µg/mL for

S. aureus and 2.0 µg/mL and 0.25 µg/mL for *P. aeruginosa*. In contrast, the MIC90 values of neomycin were 4.0 µg/mL for *S. aureus* and 16.0 µg/mL for *P. aeruginosa*. The MIC90 for polymyxin B against *P. aeruginosa* was 2.0 g/mL. These *in vitro* patterns were born out *in vivo* when microbiological eradication rates for ciprofloxacin combined with dexamethasone were superior to those for neomycin 0.35%/polymyxin B 10,000 IU/mL/hydrocortisone 1.0% otic suspension. Interestingly, OE studies with 0.3% ofloxacin used topically also found high overall bacterial eradication rates.

STEROIDS

The need for a steroid has become one of the most hotly debated issues of ototopical preparation. More study is necessary, but until better data are available, current evidence supports treating acute OE with combination steroid/antibiotic topical otic drops in most routine cases of acute OE. Thus, because the rationale for including a steroid in ototopical preparations is theoretically sound, U.S. physicians in general and otolaryngologists in particular have traditionally favored combination ototopicals that include a steroid.

Evidence Supports Steroid Use

Studies for Otitis Externa

There are convincing and supportive data to support the use of ototopicals that are steroid-containing rather than those which contain an antibiotic alone.

- One study compared the treatment of otorrhea with gentamicin alone to a colistin/neomycin/hydrocortisone combination. The authors concluded that the steroid/antibiotic combination was more effective in relieving inflammation in a shorter period of time, while gentamicin alone was more effective in eradicating the infecting organisms.
- Studies have also been done demonstrating an advantage to adding both hydrocortisone and dexamethasone to ciprofloxacin. When a combination of hydrocortisone and ciprofloxacin was used to treat patients with OE, patients with OE experienced 19 fewer hours of pain compared to those treated with ciprofloxacin alone. Although the practical significance of this finding can be debated, what is important is the proof of measurable benefit to treating OE and other infectious/inflammatory diseases of the ear with an anti-inflammatory medication.
- When neomycin 0.35%/polymyxin B 10,000 IU/mL/hydrocortisone 1.0% (N/P/H) otic suspension was compared to ciprofloxacin 0.3%/dexamethasone 0.1% (CIP/DEX) otic suspension, clinical cure rates at Day 18 were significantly higher with CIP/DEX than with N/P/H, as were microbiologic eradication rates. In addition, the clinical response was signifi-

cantly better with CIP/DEX than with N/P/H at Days 3 and 18, as was the reduction in ear inflammation at Day 18. Although study design can only allow for speculation as to why the differences were observed, one such hypothesis is that not only does the steroid confer benefit when added to an antibiotic but it may also be that the potency of the steroid matters as well. Topically in the ear, dexamethasone is likely more potent that hydrocortisone. This is discussed in greater detail below.

- Another report in 2005 demonstrated that a topical group III steroid alone was effective in treating bacterial OE caused by *P. aeruginosa* and fungal OE caused by *Candida albicans*. Although this is not to suggest that an antibiotic is not needed since studies have nicely demonstrated the need for them, this latter study should finally put to rest the question of whether or not a steroid has efficacy value in the management of OE.

Studies for Otitis Media

- In a study of 163 patients with chronic otitis media, combined gentamicin/steroid therapy was compared to placebo, and more clinical cures (52% vs. 30%) resulted with the combination.
- Several studies demonstrated that the addition of dexamethasone to a fluoroquinolone (topical ciprofloxacin/dexamethasone) compared to treatment with a quinolone alone (topical ofloxacin) resulted in advantages when treating acute otitis media with tympanostomy tubes for every outcome measured.

The relevance of these otitis media studies to the treatment of OE with a steroid/antibiotic combination is a proof-of-principal that these middle and outer ear infections are clinically defined by inflammation, and directly addressing the inflammation with anti-inflammatory medications results in improved clinical outcomes.

Additional Reasons To Include Steroids

Although formal studies show clear evidence to support the value of a steroid added to topical antibiotic formulations when treating OE, there are still other sound reasons to do so:

- To restore normal homeostatic physiology to the EAC as rapidly as possible. This is the most important reason and it cannot be overemphasized.
- To provide early, aggressive treatment to avoid complications of acute OE. These complications can include:
  - Extension beyond the confines of the EAC
  - Treatment-related emergence of resistant pathogens, secondary super-infections, loss of EAC protective measures such as down-regulation of cerumen production and increased alkalinity of EAC pH

- Transition from acute to chronic OE and
- Development of sensitization to the treatments themselves

Steroid Use in Chronic Otitis Externa

Chronic OE is also most effectively treated with a steroid-containing oto-topical agent. The data suggest that several of these cases have either no pathogen present or a sole fungal isolate.

Which Steroids To Use

Presently, several of the available steroid-containing combination ototopical agents include hydrocortisone as the anti-inflammatory agent. It is known that hydrocortisone is a relatively weak steroid when used topically. If the clinician notes an aggressive host-inflammatory response, use of a more potent steroid than hydrocortisone seems optimal until more comparative evidence becomes available.

More potent topical steroids such as dexamethasone are commercially available as ototopical FDA-approved drugs (e.g., Ciprodex® Otic), and others are currently under investigation.

OTHER THERAPIES

Systemic Antibiotics

Systemic antibiotics are those antibiotics that are delivered to the target organ via the systemic circulation. They are rarely needed (Table 4-4). Routes of administration include oral, intramuscular, intravenous, and, rarely, percutaneous and permucosal. Indications for systemic administration of antibiotics in OE include the following instances, which are discussed in detail following this list:

- In cases where OE is persistent
- In cases where there is associated otitis media

Table 4-4.
Indications for using systemic antibiotics

Persistent OE
Associated otitis media
Spread beyond the external auditory canal
High-risk patients
Early signs of necrotizing OE
Toxic state or infection unresponsive to oral antibiotics

- When local or systemic spread has occurred beyond the EAC
- In high-risk patients
- When the patient has even early signs of necrotizing OE or
- When a patient is in a toxic state or the infection is unresponsive to treatment with oral antibiotics

In cases where OE is persistent. As stated earlier, in the United States, the incidence of acute OE is cited as affecting 4/1,000/year, of which 1% (4/100,000) progresses to become chronic. These cases are particularly problematic as treatment is more challenging. Further complicating the management of chronic OE are fundamental changes in pathophysiology that, in effect, impact management. If such changes are not recognized, treatment outcomes will be compromised. These changes even affect the infectious pathogens, if indeed, some remain. It is important, therefore, to avoid applying empiric microbiologic expectations to chronic cases of OE and to avoid assuming that the pathogens responsible for the acute infection remain the same in the chronic phase. Systemic antibiotics in this condition should only be used when a culture has proven that a pathogen is present and when that pathogen is likely acting as such rather than present as a mere saprophyte. Of course, the choice of systemic agent should be based on susceptibilities and other factors known to affect pharmacokinetic and pharmacodynamic parameters.

In cases where there is associated otitis media. This is especially true in cases where the tympanic membrane is intact. The latter can occur when an otitis media episode is associated with spontaneous perforation of the tympanic membrane and secondary OE. Since the spontaneous perforation will often heal within 24 to 48 hours, the eardrum will be intact for the majority if not for the entire treatment course. Otitis media should be considered when the patient has had an upper respiratory infection or is younger than 2 years, an age when OE is uncommon.

When local or systemic spread has occurred beyond the EAC. Spread beyond the EAC should be suspected if the patient's temperature is higher than 38.3°C (101.0°F), if initial pain is severe and out of proportion to clinical findings, or if regional lymphadenopathy of the preauricular, anterior, or posterior cervical chains is present. Such instances imply more invasive infection that is "beyond the reach" of topical medications.

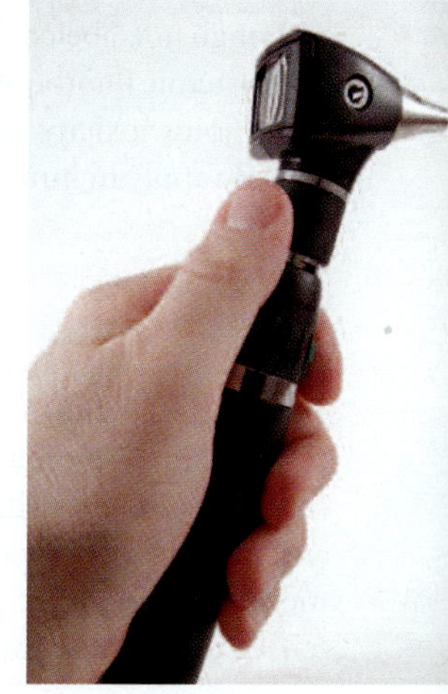

In high-risk patients. High-risk patients include diabetics, those taking systemic corticosteroids or with underlying chronic dermatitis, and the immunocompromised. These indications are more controversial since OE often resolves with topical therapy alone in these patient populations. Clearly, treatment in these cases must be individualized based on the control of the disease and the extent of the condition. A tightly controlled diabetic or an AIDS patient whose viral load is undetectable and whose T cell indices are within a favorable range can be treated more conservatively than a bone marrow transplant candidate who just underwent pre-transplant ablation. Similarly, a non-compliant patient or one who may be lost to follow-up must be managed more aggressively than one who is very compliant.

When the patient has early signs of skull base osteomyelitis. Skull base osteomyelitis can be difficult to treat and can have a high mortality rate, so providing appropriate antimicrobial therapy as soon as possible is critical.

When a patient is in a toxic state or the infection is unresponsive to treatment with oral antibiotics. This is especially true in the presence of severe pain and granulation tissue in the ear canal. In this instance, systemic parenteral antibiotics should be used. Although topical cultures may be misleading, they are recommended by some physicians to help guide treatment in such severe infections. Patients who do not respond rapidly to parenteral therapy should be referred to an otolaryngologist.

Types of Systemic Antibiotics

Whether oral or parenteral, empiric treatment should cover *Pseudomonas* and *Staphylococcus* species. This would include agents such as later generation cephalosporins, penicillinase-resistant penicillins, and fluoroquinolones. Although not labeled by the U.S. Food and Drug Administration for pediatric use, systemic fluoroquinolones seem to be safe in children. Previous concerns about joint toxicity were extrapolations from animal studies which do not directly apply to humans.

Analgesia

Often overlooked, analgesia is an important adjunct to prescribe for a patient early in the course of the disease. The analgesic used depends on the severity of the pain. Topical agents such as tetracaine and Auralgan Otic Solution® (antipyrine/benzocaine/glycerin) are commercially available for milder cases and can be especially effective at reducing ear pain in children. When pain is more severe, systemic agents such as aspirin, acetaminophen, codeine, ibuprofen, or prescription narcotics may be necessary.

As registration algorithms move more toward patient/symptom-centered outcomes and quality of care measures become increasingly more important, pain relief intervention is clearly the most obvious to the patient and the most direct contributor to patient satisfaction. As was discussed in Chapter 4, pain relief is achieved more rapidly when an anti-inflammatory agent is added to an antibiotic in combination ototopical preparations. Pain in this condition is usually directly related to *inflammation* and reinforces the importance of addressing inflammation directly when making treatment choices.

Acidification

Acidification is sometimes used to either maintain physiologic acid pH in the EAC if cerumen is not being normally produced or as prophylaxis in recurrent cases. This is especially true in patients with risk factors such as swimming that alter the physiologic pH of the EAC. Further, acidification is known to be an effective treatment for OE as evidenced by studies with acetic acid.

Agents whose active ingredient is acid alone have several disadvantages that affect both patient compliance and safety. What is less certain is whether agents with other active ingredients that are also acidic are more effective than those that are not. This author is unaware of any controlled, prospective, randomized, and blinded studies controlled for this factor alone. Nevertheless, even in the absence of such data, it appears logical that agents that directly treat the infection and inflammation while at the same time work toward restoring physiologic pH are ideal.

Ear Candling

One approach to treating OE, called ear candling, has been used for nearly 1,000 years in many diverse geographic locations, including North America, South America, China, and Egypt. This therapy involves placing a hollow candle into the EAC and lighting the opposite end, which is thought to create a vacuum that draws cerumen, bacteria, and debris out of the ear (Figure 4-1). One can find ear candles on the shelves of many retail stores as they are still used today by holistic and alternative health practitioners.

Unfortunately, results from a clinical study suggest that this procedure is not effective and might actually be harmful. The study examined the ability of commercially available ear candles to generate a vacuum and to remove

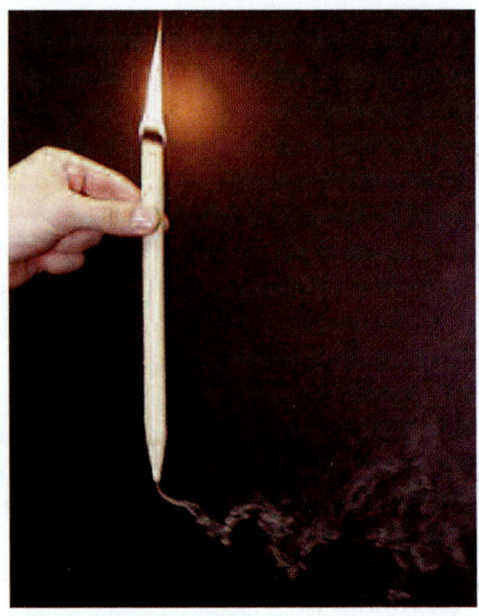

Figure 4-1. Ear candle. This therapy involves placing a hollow candle into the external ear canal and lighting the opposite end, which is thought to create a vacuum that draws cerumen, bacteria, and debris out of the ear. At least one study suggests that ear candling is not effective and might be harmful. Accessed at: http://altmed.creighton.edu/ear/experiment.htm

cerumen from eight ears; four of the eight ears had impacted cerumen. After 20 attempts with two different candle types, the generation of a vacuum could not be demonstrated with a device consisting of a 2-chambered tube with a tympanometer probe inside each chamber. The ear candles also did not remove any noticeable cerumen from the four impacted ears, and the procedure actually deposited candle wax in two of the four ears that were originally free of excess cerumen. Interestingly, results from a survey of otolaryngologists conducted by the authors revealed that one third of the responding physicians were aware of ear candling by one or more of their patients. In addition, 21 ear injuries were reported among 20 patients who were treated by these physicians for ear candle-induced complications. These injuries included burns, occlusions of the ear canal with candle wax, and a tympanic membrane perforation.

Topical Astringents and Alcohols

The topical application of various astringents and alcohols has been used throughout history for ear infections. Those preparations that were acidic or contained high concentrations of alcohol may have been effective if they were administered early in the disease. In fact, certain astringents, such as boric acid and aluminum acetate, are considered effective and are sometimes used today. The disadvantages of using these treatments are that they may not have adequate antimicrobial activity to eradicate pathogens in moderate-to-severe cases and they can be painful to the patient, which may affect compliance. Safety is of particular concern in the instance of a non-intact tympanic membrane.

Surgery

Surgery is rarely required for cases of OE, but may be necessary in cases of necrotizing OE wherein devitalized sequestrations of bone may need to be debrided. The surgical management of necrotizing OE is discussed in Chapter 6.

Surgery may also be needed in cases of a very narrow EAC secondary to grossly hypertrophic canal skin.

Swimmer's osteomas can predispose to OE and may require surgical removal.

SUMMARY

The vast majority of cases of OE respond to aural toilet and the application of topical therapy, generally steroid/antibiotic drops. Several types of therapies exist, but topical therapy has many advantages, not the least of which is that the medication is delivered directly to the target organ. At this time, the only FDA-approved combination topical agent that is proven to be effective and safe if the integrity of the tympanic membrane is in question is ciprofloxacin/dexamethasone (Ciprodex® Otic) (Figure 4-2). Systemic antibiotics should be used if the OE is spreading or when medically indicated. If symptoms persist, obtain a culture and change therapy accordingly. When there is no improvement, patients should be referred to a specialist.

Evidence-based recommendations exist for the management of diffuse acute OE, the most common form of OE. These recommendations can guide many uncomplicated management decisions.

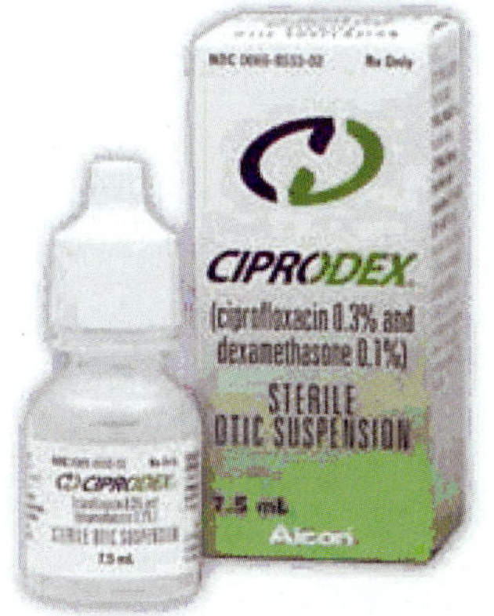

Figure 4-2. Ciprodex® Otic. At this time, Ciprodex® Otic is the only FDA-approved combination topical agent that would be effective and safe if the integrity of the tympanic membrane is in question. Accessed at: http://www.ciprodex.com/consumer/CIPRODEX_Otic.asp

5

Prevention

We must not forget the great tendency to recurrence.
—Dr. R. F. Harrell,
The New Orleans Medical and Surgical Journal, 1908

PDQ fact: *Preventing the occurrence—or recurrence—of otitis externa primarily consists of avoiding predisposing factors and treating underlying dermatological conditions.*

Preventing the occurrence—or recurrence—of OE primarily consists of avoiding predisposing factors and treating underlying dermatological conditions (Table 5-1).

Table 5-1.
Tips for preventing otitis externa

- Avoiding swimming until infection resolves—institute dry ear precautions thereafter
- Reducing trauma to the external auditory canal—scratching or overzealous cleaning
- Using acidifying drops—helps restore acidic pH to the external auditory canal
- Using astringents—but these may burn and sting and are not often used

PROVIDING TIPS TO SWIMMERS

Swimming should be avoided until the infection resolves and, when swimming resumes, dry ear precautions should be instituted. This cannot be emphasized enough. Swimming too soon adversely affects outcomes in two ways:

- It potentially introduces additional pathogens into the ear canal, already compromised by active or resolving infection and

- It perpetuates the abnormal physiology that set the stage for the infection in the first place

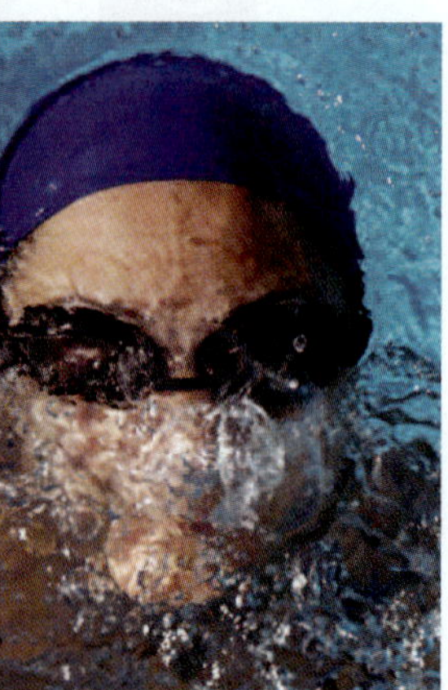

Examples of the latter circumstance are increases in pH and continued removal of protective host defenses such as cerumen.

The following tips for protection against OE should be offered to all swimmers:

Dry ears after swimming. Those who find it difficult to get water out of the ears should apply a few drops of an alcohol-based ear product into the ear. Such products are commercially available at most local drug stores as over-the-counter preparations. These preparations should only be considered in healthy ears that are producing cerumen and that are completely normal with intact tympanic membranes.

Know a pool's chlorine and pH testing program. One can ask a pool manager or, in the case of those who own a pool, pay meticulous attention to these details. Pool chemistry can fluctuate significantly and relatively little time is needed for pathogens to proliferate within them. Although the primary mechanism underlying swimming as it relates to OE is not the direct introduction of pathogens into the EAC, water source-related outbreaks of OE have been documented. Pools and hot tubs with good chemistry and pH control are less likely to spread OE.

Avoid polluted water. Swimmers should pay attention to signage and avoid swimming in locations that have been closed because of pollution.

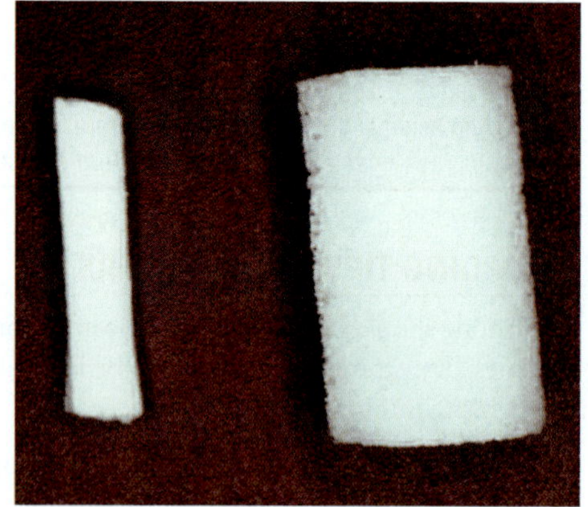

Early acute diffuse otitis externa (swimmer's ear). Acute diffuse otitis externa (swimmer's ear) is an acute, diffuse, painful bacterial infection of the skin of the external auditory canal. The chief agents responsible for the development of acute diffuse otitis externa are local trauma and moisture. Gram-negative bacteria, principally *Pseudomonas aeruginosa*, can be cultured in most cases. The skin of the external canal is swollen, extremely tender, and shiny. Severe pain is usually present.

Avoid putting objects in the ear. Items such as fingers or cotton swabs and in the case of swimmers—ear plugs—can scratch the EAC and provide a site for infection.

REDUCING TRAUMA TO THE EXTERNAL AUDITORY CANAL

Trauma to the EAC can be caused by scratching or overzealous cleaning. Thereafter, the inflamed skin often causes microscopic breaches in the integrity of the epithelium. Naturally, the flora in patients with OE often includes pathogens not typically present in healthy ear canals. These microscopic breaks within the epithelium serve as portals of entry for these pathogens into the deeper levels of the skin lining the EAC and thus allow for the development of acute OE.

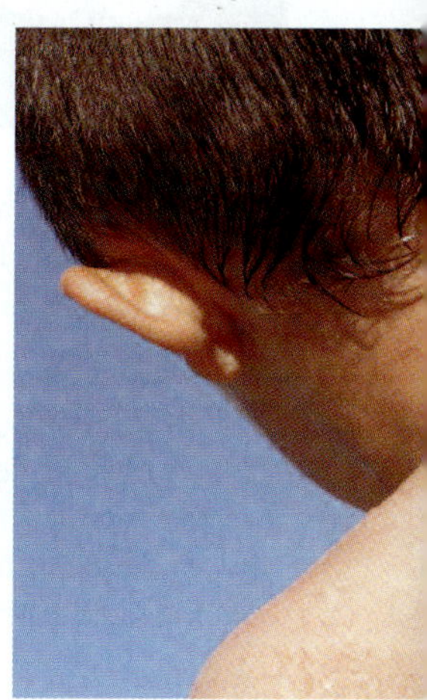

It has been shown in dermatology that steroids can reverse some or all of these epithelial changes and, thus, reduce the incidence of secondary infections. If topical steroids alone fail, consideration should be given to a short course of systemic steroids. This may seem contrary to what one would ideally choose since steroids are known immunosuppressive drugs, but this side effect is not seen in short-course systemic therapy. Additionally, topical steroids may be of considerable benefit in reducing residual pruritus. Although not definitively proven, it is also likely that topical steroids are of benefit in preventing acute exacerbation of OE in patients with chronic OE.

USING ACIDIFYING DROPS

Acidifying drops may be beneficial. Not only do these drops restore acidic pH to the EAC but they are also bactericidal as a result of both the active and often the inactive ingredients in the formulations. Many have suggested that the ideal prophylactic is a combination of both an acidifying and a drying agent.

PDQ fact: *The ideal prophylactic for otitis externa is likely a combination of both an acidifying and a drying agent.*

Experiences with Divers

Saturation divers spend up to a month in diving chambers aboard ships. There, they are kept at the same depth as the job they are performing in the

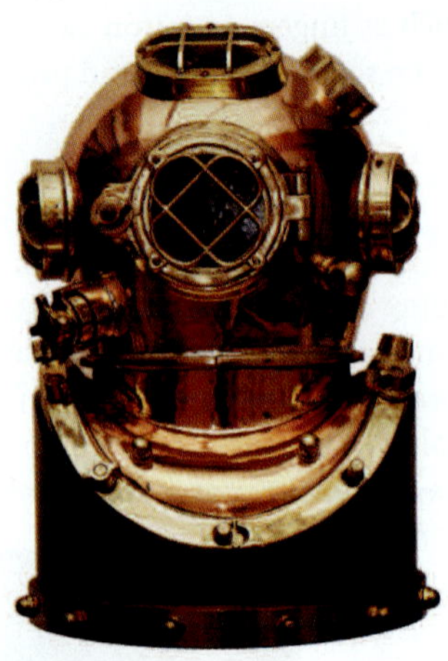

sea, whether it's salvaging a sunken vessel or performing a research project. Each day these divers are transferred from the chamber to the work site in a diving bell. The divers spend a great deal of their time immersed. Both the chamber and the bell provide a hot, humid environment that is perfect for breaking down the cellular lining of the ear canal; the result is often OE. As one might presume, such circumstances represent the extreme in terms of risk for developing recurrent OE. Rates as high as 20% have been reported. Otic Domeboro® Solution, which is 2% acetic acid, water, aluminum acetate, sodium acetate, and boric acid, is one example of a preparation that contains both an acidifying and a drying agent. This external ear prophylaxis remains a standard part of U.S. Navy Saturation diving procedure. The U.S. Navy Diving Manual States:

The head is tilted to one side and the external ear canal gently filled with the solution, which must remain in the canal for five minutes. The head is then tilted to the other side, the solution allowed to run out, and the procedure repeated for the other ear. The five-minute duration must be timed with a watch. If the solution does not remain in the ear a full five minutes, the effectiveness of the procedure is greatly reduced.

Acidifying drops are useful for sport diving, too, when there are frequent dives over several days. The acid retards bacterial growth, while the aluminum and sodium acetate act as astringents (discussed in the next section), drawing excess water out of the cells lining the ear canal. Reports state that such preparations effectively prevent OE only if they remain in the EAC for five minutes. Shorter resident time was unsuccessful. Similarly, longer resident time for ototopicals in the EAC as well as in the middle ear (in the range of five minutes) has been shown to improve treatment outcomes. Although no clinical trials compare resident times as the sole independent variable, indirect support from pharmacokinetic and pharmacodynamic modeling would strongly support this concept and this is likely one of the mechanisms by which otowicks (described in Chapter 4) improve cure rates.

USING ASTRINGENTS

Before antibiotic availability, the mainstay of treatment of OE was topical compounds containing astringents such as aluminum acetate solutions (Burow's

Solution USP, Otic Domeboro®, and others) and acetic acid solutions (Vosol Otic). These preparations are still widely used but principally to *prevent* OE.

In one study, topical 8% aluminum acetate solution was as effective as a commonly used antimicrobial-corticosteroid topical mixture (polymyxin/neomycin/hydrocortisone) for 25 adult patients with OE (72% vs. 76%, respectively). In a double-blind, randomized study involving 65 adults and children, the effectiveness of aluminum acetate equaled that of gentamicin solution. In a Dutch study evaluating OE in 213 adults, topical antibiotics were more effective than topical acetic acid alone and alleviated symptoms faster than acetic acid plus steroids.

Unfortunately, there is a lack of high-quality published trials, which defaults evidence-based decision-making to provider experience and patient preference. In this regard, topical astringents often sting and burn upon instillation, adverse effects that significantly increase non-compliance with therapy. Other than prevention of OE, practitioners usually reserve nonspecific therapy such as acetic acid and Burow's solution for self-medication and for mild symptoms. Studies that include measures of clinical goals, such as pain relief, cessation of symptoms, and eradication of infection are needed before astringent agents can be recommended for routine therapy of moderate to severe OE. Most treatment data concerning OE have centered on therapy with antimicrobial otic drops alone or combined with a steroid.

SUMMARY

If OE is present, those who swim should avoid this activity until the infection resolves. For all swimmers, dry ear precautions should be recommended. If OE is present (and even if it is not), discourage scratching or overzealous cleaning of the EAC as microscopic breaches in epithelium can permit pathogens to enter. Some suggest that the ideal prophylactic to OE is a combination acidifying/drying agent. Astringents can be of some benefit but since they burn or sting upon installation, patient compliance can be low.

FLASHBACK

One hundred years ago, more than 95% of all U.S. doctors had no college education. Instead, they attended so-called medical schools, many of which were condemned in the press and by the government as substandard.

6

Other Types of OE Diagnosis and Management

While in many of these cases the disease seems very mild and of little consequence, yet we should in all cases remember the possibility of grave and even fatal termination.

—Dr. R. F. Harrell,
The New Orleans Medical and Surgical Journal, 1908

ACUTE LOCALIZED (CIRCUMSCRIBED) OTITIS EXTERNA (FURUNCULOSIS)

Acute localized (circumscribed) otitis externa, also called *furunculosis,* is often considered a complication of OE.

Signs and Symptoms

Acute localized (circumscribed) OE is characterized by distinct areas of inflammation that may include blister-like swellings. Localized swelling is usually significant and may include a superficial abscess that can be drained. One form, usually Gram-positive and commonly caused by *Staphylococcus aureus,* forms in one or more hair follicles in the ear canal. This can result in the development of severe inflammation surrounding the follicle, sometimes referred to as a furuncle, or boil (Figure 6-1).

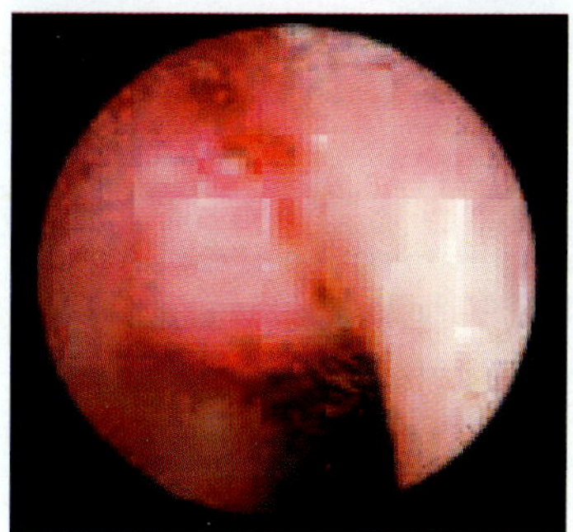

Figure 6-1. **Furuncle.** This shows severe inflammation surrounding the follicle, sometimes referred to as a boil.

Etiology

Generally, a focal furuncle of the lateral third of the EAC occurs as a result of obstructed apopilosebaceous glands.

Treatment

Patients are treated with local heat, ototopical antibiotics combined with steroid, and systemic antibiotics in the inflammatory stage. This disease often progresses or presents as an abscess that may require surgical incision and drainage if it fails conservative medical therapy.

ECZEMATOUS OTITIS EXTERNA (DERMATITIC OTITIS EXTERNA)

Eczematous otitis externa, sometimes referred to as *dermatitic otitis externa*, encompasses various dermatologic conditions (e.g., atopic dermatitis, psoriasis lupus erythematous, and eczema) that may affect the EAC (Figure 6-2).

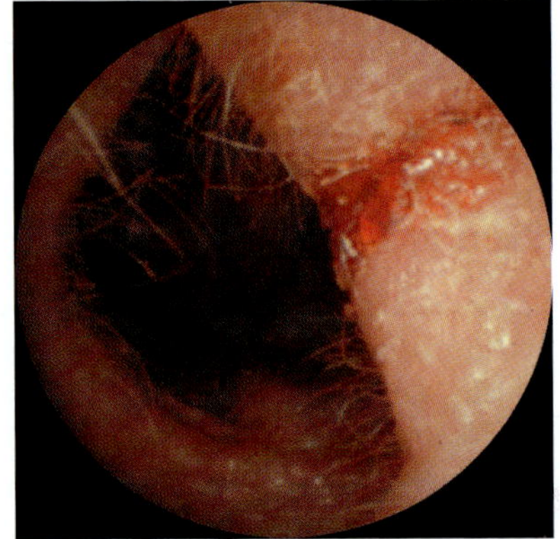

Figure 6-2. External canal seborrheic dermatitis. This view shows long-standing seborrhea with recurrent pruritus of the external canal. The canal wall is dry and scaly with excoriation.

Signs and Symptoms

A chronic, persistent low-grade infection and inflammation of the EAC may comprise the presentation. In these cases, the EAC lacks cerumen and is lined by dry, hypertrophic skin with variable swelling and stenosis (Figure 6-3). Mucopurulent otorrhea and excoriated skin may also be present.

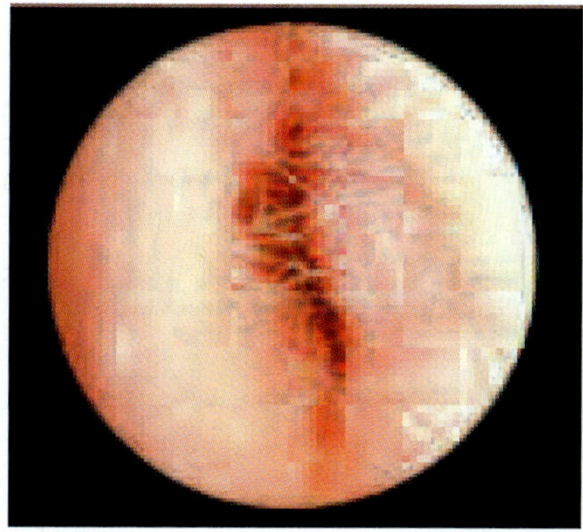

Figure 6-3. Chronic otitis externa with canal skin hypertrophy. In these cases, the external ear canal lacks cerumen and is lined by dry, hypertrophic skin with variable swelling and stenosis.

If there are lesions, they typically occur in the ear canal and elsewhere on the body, especially the head and neck. At a minimum, involvement of the skin of the auricle is seen in most cases, at least at the level of the external auditory meatus and conchal bowl. This is rare in most cases of acute diffuse OE and in circumscript OE.

Manifestations in the EAC can range from mild erythema and scaling with atopic dermatitis, to dense, adherent scaling with psoriasis, to the focal inflammatory changes of acne. Pruritus is the most common symptom.

Diagnosis

It is critical to inspect skin throughout the patient as this markedly improves the likelihood of an accurate diagnosis and increases the likelihood of a successful treatment outcome.

Often the most challenging diagnostic dilemma of eczematous OE is what this author calls "the chicken-egg" debate. On the one hand, eczema of the EAC skin may occur as a primary diagnosis. Although many specific skin conditions are possible, seborrhea, psoriasis, and acne vulgaris are just a few examples of common primary dermatologic conditions that may affect the EAC. In such cases, this underlying primary condition may predispose to secondary infection and attention to treatment of both is critical for complete cure and for prevention of recurrence.

PDQ fact: *Dermatologic conditions of the external auditory canal skin may occur as a result of either incompletely treated otitis externa or of the treatments themselves.*

Etiology

Dermatologic conditions of the EAC skin may occur *as a result of* either incompletely treated OE or of the treatments themselves. Thus, the causative bacteria vary greatly because many of the patients have already received prolonged topical therapy. At times, only normal flora can be cultured. This points out why it is so critical to aggressively treat OE in its acute phase. This has been emphasized in other places in this book but is so important that it deserves repetition.

There is often a family history and a recurrent course.

Treatment

Treatment consists of the use of acidifying drops combined with steroid drops, but persistent cases require referral to an otolaryngologist for frequent otomicroscopic cleansing and debridement. Rarely, surgery is needed to enlarge and resurface the EAC.

Treatment also involves addressing the infectious cause as well as the inflammatory consequence of the infection. As to the latter, certain treatments, especially topical ones such as neomycin or thimerosal-containing drops, may themselves promote a host inflammatory reaction and, thus, lead to secondary dermatologic disease. Though tempting to dismiss this as "academic jabberwocky," the practical importance of such determinations cannot be emphasized enough.

ID REACTION (AUTOECZEMATIZATION)[1]

Id reaction (autoeczematization) is a generalized acute cutaneous reaction to a variety of stimuli, including infectious and inflammatory skin conditions. The pruritic rash that characterizes the id reaction has been referred to as dermatophytid, pediculid, or bacterid when associated with a corresponding infectious process.

Signs and Symptoms

Dermatological manifestations vary and depend on the etiology of the eruption. General history may include the following:

- Varying degrees of pruritus
- An acute onset of an extremely pruritic, erythematous, maculopapular, or papulovesicular eruption 1-2 weeks after primary infection or dermatitis
- Exacerbation of the preexisting dermatitis induced by infection, scratching, or inappropriate therapy (Id reaction to tinea incognito has been reported)

- Dermatological manifestation subsequent to radiation treatment for tinea capitis
- Vesicles on the hands or feet
- Tenderness in the fingers
- Clinical lesions of id reactions are variable and are largely predicated on the inciting etiology. Lesions are, by definition, at a site distant from the primary infection or dermatitis. They are usually distributed symmetrically.
- A widespread, symmetrical eruption of small follicular papules associated with a kerion and a pompholyxlike eruption are usually associated with inflammatory tinea pedis (common)
- An acute, intensely pruritic, symmetric maculopapular or papulovesicular reaction that involves the forearms, thighs, legs, trunk, face, hands, neck, and feet (in descending order of frequency) is typical of the id reaction with stasis dermatitis (common)
- Erysipelaslike eruption on the anterior leg secondary to a dermatophytosis may occur (less common)
- Extracutaneous manifestations include fever, anorexia, generalized adenopathy, splenomegaly, and leukocytosis (uncommon)
- The clinical picture can mimic erythema multiforme (rare)

Diagnosis

Laboratory workup of id reactions is clearly indicated for dermatophytids. Absence of fungi in the dermatophytid lesions and clearing of the dermatophytid after the fungus is eradicated are necessary to confirm a definitive diagnosis of a dermatophytid reaction.

Strict criteria include a proven dermatophyte infection and a positive skin test finding for a group-specific trichophytin antigen.

All too frequently, the focus is on the presenting complaint. In the case of OE, doing a complete body examination is often not considered. Yet, it is

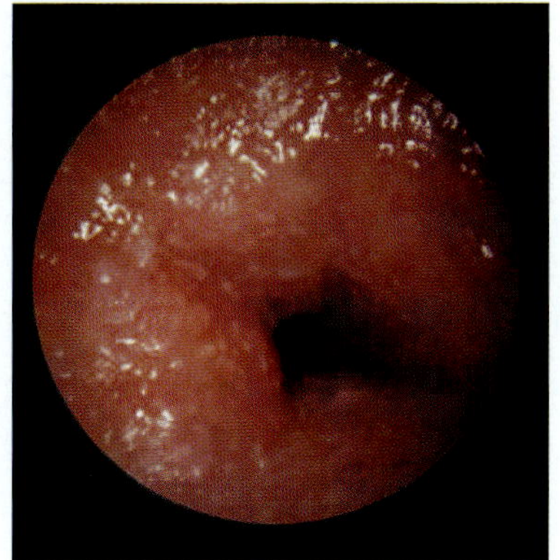

Acute allergic otitis externa: neomycin contact dermatitis. In refractory cases of acute and chronic otitis externa, the examiner should be on the look-out for allergic reactions to the medications used, eg, neomycin contact dermatitis. The possibility of an underlying dermatologic disorder, systemic disease, or even malignancy must always be considered in unresponsive cases.

not infrequent that a fungal infection in between the toes is the nidus of a recurrent id reaction in the EAC. Even in cases where a full body examination is performed, it is easy to overlook a pathophysiologic link between a fungal foot infection and OE.

PDQ fact: *In the case of otitis externa, doing a complete body examination is often not considered. Yet, it is not infrequent that a fungal infection in between the toes is the nidus of a recurrent id reaction in the external auditory canal.*

Etiology

While the exact cause of the id reaction is unknown, the following factors are thought to be responsible:

- Abnormal immune recognition of autologous skin antigens
- Increased stimulation of normal T cells by altered skin constituents
- Lowering of the irritation threshold
- Dissemination of infectious antigen with a secondary response and
- Hematogenous dissemination of cytokines from a primary site

Id reactions result from a variety of stimuli, including infectious entities and inflammatory skin conditions:

- Infections with dermatophytes, pulmonary histoplasmosis, mycobacteria, viruses, bacteria, or parasites (pediculosis)
- Contact dermatitis, stasis dermatitis, or other eczematous dermatoses

Papulonecrotic tuberculid, and some other tuberculids, are now thought to be true cutaneous forms of tuberculosis and not id reactions because of the identification (by polymerase chain reaction) of *Mycobacterium tuberculosis* in lesions.

Treatment

The goal is to adequately treat the primary infection or dermatitis. Fortunately, this will lead to prompt resolution of the id reaction regardless of the mechanism. Recurrences are common, especially if the primary source is not treated adequately. Treatment of eruption should include:

- Systemic or topical corticosteroids
- Wet compresses
- Systemic or topical antihistamines

OTOMYCOSIS (FUNGAL OTITIS EXTERNA)

Otomycosis (fungal otitis externa) is a superficial infection of the EAC most often characterized by inflammation, pruritus, scaling, and severe discomfort.

Signs and Symptoms

When symptoms are present, discomfort is the most common complaint, primarily taking the form of pruritus and a feeling of fullness in the ear. Pruritus may be quite intense, resulting in scratching and further damage to the epidermis.

Diagnosis

Since otomycosis is often associated with mild symptoms, observing the unique discharge in the EAC often makes the diagnosis. This discharge is typically fluffy and white, but may also be black, gray, bluish-green, or yellow (Figure 6-4). It can also present as black or white conidiophores on white hyphae associated with *Aspergillus* (Figure 6-5).

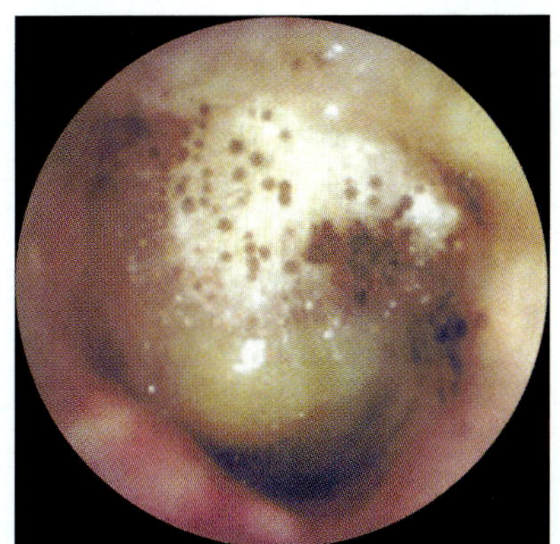

Figure 6-4. Otomycosis. The white, cotton-like material with small black tufts in this ear canal represents topical fungal infection, or fungal otitis externa. This may occur in humid environments or when the ear canal has been topically treated with antibiotic eardrops.

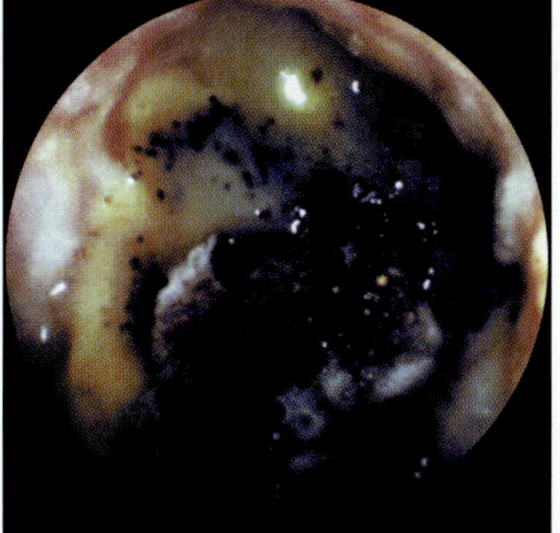

Figure 6-5. Otomycosis. Exudate and black mycelia are seen in this case of external otitis due to *Aspergillus niger*.

Fungi in the ear can behave similar to the spectrum of fungal disease in the paranasal sinuses. Specifically, they may be present as saprophytes or may cause invasive non-fulminant and invasive fulminant disease. Also, there is increasing evidence that allergic fungal otitis is a distinct and real entity conferring yet another potential role for fungi in OE. Making these diagnostic distinctions is crucial to treatment.

PDQ fact: *In no other type of otitis externa than in otomycosis is it more important to focus treatment on restoration of normal physiologic pH.*

Etiology

The most common pathogen is *Aspergillus* (80-90% of cases are from *A. niger, A. flavus, A. fumigatus*), followed by *Candida albicans*. Other more rare fungal pathogens include *Phycomycetes, Rhizopus, Actinomyces,* and *Penicillium*. As fungal isolation techniques become more sophisticated, it is likely that several other species will be identified in OE.

Classically, otomycosis may result from prolonged bacterial OE that renders the EAC vulnerable to opportunistic infection such as yeast or mold. Mixed bacterial and fungal infections are thus common. However, fungus is occasionally the primary pathogen in OE, especially in the presence of excessive moisture or heat.

Treatment

Uncomplicated cases of otomycosis may also be treated with antifungal drops. Lotrimin drops are effective in cases where the tympanic membrane is known to be intact.

However, fungal OE can be one of the most challenging entities to treat. In no other type of OE than in otomycosis is it more important to focus treatment on restoration of normal physiologic pH. Aggressive aural toilet is paramount. As is true of most fungal infections, mechanical removal of as much fungus as possible is crucial. This also reduces moisture within the EAC. At times, aural toilet alone is all that is needed. Other times, antifungal powders provide the triple benefits of drying, antifungal activity, and in the case of those that also contain an acid such as boric acid, acidification. There are also combination powders available that contain not only an antifungal and acidifying agent but also an antibacterial agent if bacteria are acting as co-pathogens.

In the case of invasive fungal disease, at a minimum, systemic antifungal azole derivatives (i.e., fluconazole) are needed. Rarely, surgical debridement and possibly even a lateral temporal bone resection may be necessary in cases where the patient is markedly immunocompromised and where the middle-ear cleft, EAC, and beyond are involved. Similarly, those patients with a fungal id reaction in the EAC must have the primary skin fungal source identified and treated along with the EAC. These patients may also require systemic antifungal treatment as certain fungal infections, such as those affecting the nail beds, may be too deeply invasive to be managed with topical therapy.

Patients with allergic fungal otitis may require not only systemic antifungal therapy but also desensitization immunotherapy. Specific skin testing in conjunction with an allergist experienced in treating this condition is very helpful.

HERPES ZOSTER OTICUS[2]

Herpes zoster oticus is a viral infection caused by varicella zoster. If there is a reactivation of the varicella-zoster virus along the distribution of the sensory nerves innervating the ear, which usually includes the geniculate ganglion of the facial nerve, Ramsay Hunt syndrome occurs as a result (Figure 6-6).

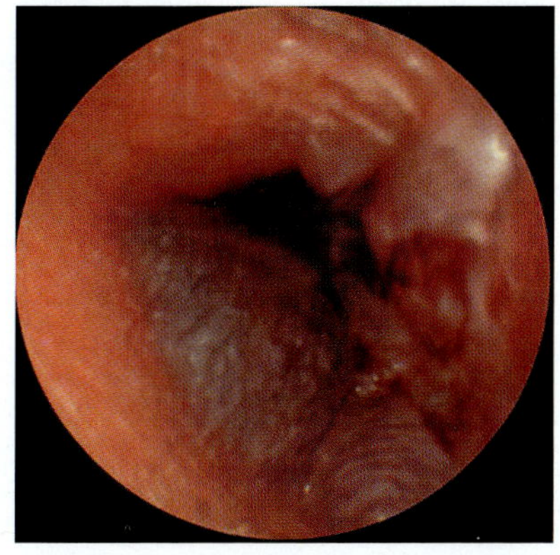

Figure 6-6. Herpes zoster oticus. Herpes zoster oticus (Ramsay Hunt syndrome) is a herpes zoster infection of the seventh cranial nerve. Here, vesicles are seen involving the medial ear canal and tympanic membrane.

Signs and Symptoms

Herpes zoster manifests as a vesicular rash, usually in a single dermatome. Most patients who develop the condition have a 2-3 day prodrome of pain, tingling, or burning in the involved dermatome. It is during the prodrome that misdiagnosis is most likely. During this prodromal period, patients may present with symptoms consistent with acute myocardial infarction, urolithiasis, pleurisy, trigeminal neuralgia, appendicitis, cholelithiasis, or herniated nucleus pulposus with radiculopathy, depending upon the involved dermatome. The most commonly involved dermatomes are of the thorax. Development of the rash may be preceded by paresthesias or pain along the involved dermatome. Ocular involvement and zoster keratitis may result if reactivation occurs along the ophthalmic division of the trigeminal nerve.

Ramsay Hunt syndrome type I is characterized by intense ear otalgia, a rash around the ear, mouth, face, neck, and scalp, and paralysis of facial nerves. Other symptoms may include hearing loss, vertigo, and tinnitus. Taste loss in the tongue and dry mouth and eyes may also occur. Occasionally, Ramsay Hunt syndrome is associated with vertigo, tinnitus, and hearing disorders.

Diagnosis

Diagnosis of herpes zoster is based primarily on clinical findings. In some patients, the presentation of herpes zoster can be atypical and may require additional testing. This is particularly true in immunocompromised patients.

Varicella-zoster virus can be cultured successfully; however, this method is not practical for use in the emergency department because of the virus' slow growth. Tzanck smear can be obtained from the vesicular lesions; however, the smear does not differentiate between varicella-zoster virus infections such as herpes zoster and herpes simplex. Direct immunofluorescence assay may be performed to detect varicella-zoster and can distinguish varicella-zoster from herpes simplex.

Other tests and procedures can be used for diagnosis but are less common. They include monoclonal antibody tests and blood mononuclear cell testing for viral DNA (for research purposes). Biopsy for direct immunofluorescence testing is rarely performed.

PDQ fact: The incidence of herpes zoster oticus increases significantly in patients older than 60 years.

Etiology

Varicella-zoster virus infection initially produces chickenpox. Following resolution of the chickenpox, the virus lies dormant in the dorsal root ganglia until focal reactivation along a ganglion's distribution results in herpes zoster (shingles). Although the exact precipitants that result in viral reactivation are not known certainly, decreased cellular immunity appears to increase the risk of reactivation.

Incidence

The incidence of herpes zoster oticus increases significantly in patients older than 60 years. Approximately 95% of adults in the United States have antibodies to the varicella-zoster virus. The incidence is equal in males and females and increases with age. Among those patients who have had exposure to chickenpox, blacks are 25% less likely than whites to develop herpes zoster. Approximately 80% of cases occur in persons older than 20 years. Herpes zoster occurs annually in 300,000-500,000 individuals and this year it is expected that more than one million Americans will develop shingles.

Ramsay Hunt syndrome is a relatively common complication of shingles and accounts for up to 12% of all facial paralyses in the United States.

Complications

Herpes Zoster

- **Postherpetic neuralgia.** This is a common complication, characterized by pain that persists for longer than 1 month following resolution of the vesicular rash. This complication is more common in patients older than 50 years. Postherpetic neuralgia may develop as a continuation of pain that accompanies acute zoster or it may develop following apparent resolution of the initial zoster reactivation. The pain of postherpetic neuralgia usually resolves within 6 months. However, 1% of patients continue to have pain for 1 year or longer.
- **Superinfection of skin lesions.** Herpes zoster may be associated with a secondary bacterial infection (typically streptococcal or staphylococcal) of the vesicular rash.

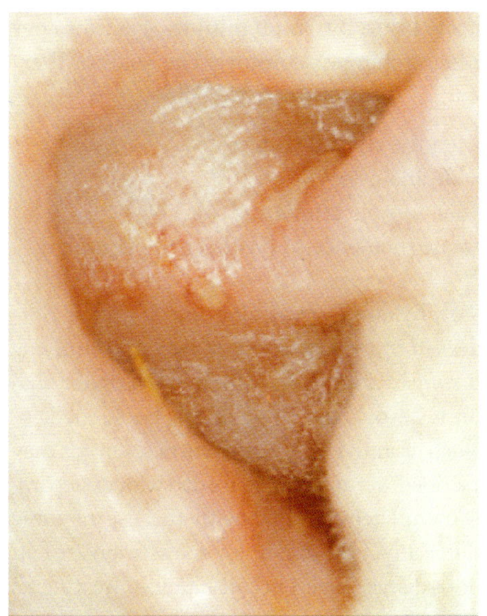

Herpes zoster oticus (Ramsay Hunt syndrome). Herpes zoster oticus is a viral infection of the geniculate ganglion (seventh cranial nerve), characterized by a vesicular eruption of the skin of the external ear. Herpes zoster oticus may also be associated with a herpes infection of the upper cervical roots or the glossopharyngeal nerve, the latter producing vesicles on the soft palate. Initially, the patient experiences a hot feeling within the ear, which rapidly develops into pain of increasing severity. Hearing loss, tinnitus, or vertigo may be present when the inner ear is involved and facial paralysis if the facial nerve is involved. Note the characteristic vesicles on the conchal bowl.

- **Ocular involvement.** Herpes zoster involving the second branch of the trigeminal nerve may be associated with conjunctivitis, keratitis, corneal ulceration, iridocyclitis, glaucoma, and blindness.
- **Meningoencephalitis and other central nervous system complications.** Meningoencephalitis secondary to herpes zoster is more likely to be seen in immunocompromised patients than in immunocompetent patients. Other central nervous system complications may include myelitis, cranial nerve palsies, and granulomatous angiitis. Granulomatous angiitis may result in the development of a cerebrovascular accident.
- **Disseminated zoster in immunocompromised patients.** In such cases, hematogenous spread may result in the involvement of multiple dermatomes. Visceral involvement also can occur. Such systemic involvement can lead to death due to encephalitis, hepatitis, or pneumonitis.

Ramsay-Hunt Syndrome

- Peripheral facial nerve weakness and deafness
- Cranial nerve syndromes, particularly ophthalmic and facial
- Guillain-Barré syndrome

Treatment

Most cases are self-limited and require only treatment of the symptoms. NSAIDs have been quite useful for pain control and only rarely are narcotics needed. Wet dressings with tap water or 5% aluminum acetate (Burow's solution) should be applied to the affected skin for 30-60 minutes 4-6 times per day. Lotions (i.e., calamine) may help relieve discomfort. The goals of therapy in herpes zoster infection are to:

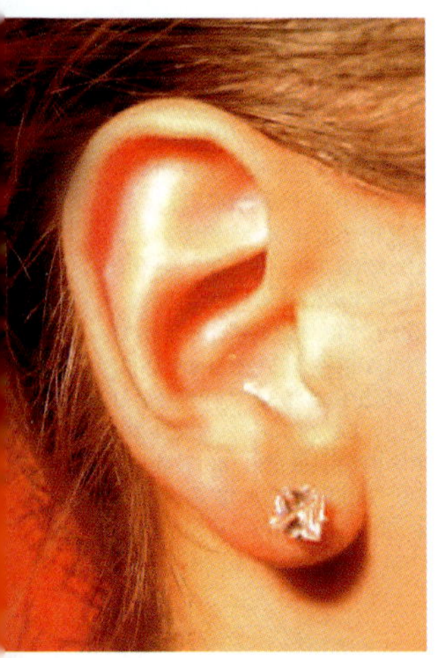

- Shorten the clinical course
- Provide analgesia
- Prevent complications and
- Decrease incidence of postherpetic neuralgia

Use of steroid-containing antibiotics is contraindicated in viral infections of the EAC, including herpes simplex infections. Although a detailed discussion is beyond the scope of this book, medications such as antiviral drugs or corticosteroids may be prescribed. Vertigo may be treated with diazepam. If not completely familiar with the use of these drugs, it is advisable to employ the assistance of an infectious disease expert in consultation. Treatments are summarized in Table 6-1.

Table 6-1.

Treatment for herpes zoster oticus

Antiviral agents—Acyclovir antivirals may decrease incidence of postherpetic neuralgia. Famciclovir and valacyclovir (two antiviral agents with properties similar to those of acyclovir) offer better dosing regimens than acyclovir and yet are less studied.

Drug Name	Indications	Dosing
Acyclovir (Zovirax®)	Reduces duration of symptomatic lesions. Indicated for patients presenting within 48-72 h of onset of rash. Treated patients experience less pain and faster resolution of cutaneous lesions.	*Adult:* Immunocompromised adults: 800 mg PO q4h (5 times/d) for 7-10 d; alternatively, 10 mg/kg/dose or 500 mg/m²/dose IV q8h. *Pediatric:* Immunocompromised children: 250-600 mg/m²/dose PO 4-5 times/d for 7-10 d; alternatively, 10 mg/kg/dose or 500 mg/m²/dose IV q8h
Famciclovir (Famvir®)	Prodrug that, when biotransformed into active metabolite penciclovir, may inhibit viral DNA synthesis/replication.	*Adult:* 500 mg PO q8h for 7 d. *Pediatric:* Not established
Valacyclovir (Valtrex®)	Prodrug rapidly converted to acyclovir before exerting its antiviral activity. More expensive but more convenient dosing regimen than acyclovir.	*Adult:* 1000 mg PO q8h for 7 d. *Pediatric:* Limited information available: 30 mg/kg/dose PO q8h or 7 days (per Pediatric Dosage Handbook, 13th ed.)

Corticosteroids—These agents have anti-inflammatory properties and cause profound and varied metabolic effects. Corticosteroids modify the body's immune response to diverse stimuli.

Drug Name	Indications	Dosing
Prednisone (Deltasone®, Orasone®, Meticorten®)	The addition of a corticosteroid to acyclovir resulted in decreased acute pain but no decrease in long-term pain. One study also demonstrated more rapid initial healing of rash, although time to complete rash resolution was unchanged.	*Adult:* 60 mg/d PO for 4-5 days, then tapered over 3 wk. *Pediatric:* 0.05-2 mg/kg PO divided bid/qid for 3-5 days, then tapered over 2 wk

Analgesics—Pain control is essential to quality patient care. Analgesics ensure patient comfort, promote pulmonary toilet, and enable physical therapy regimens. Most analgesics have sedating properties that are beneficial for patients who have skin lesions.

Drug Name	Indication	Dosing
Acetaminophen (Tylenol®, Aspirin-Free Anacin®)	Drug of choice for treatment of pain in patients who (1) have documented hypersensitivity to aspirin or NSAIDs; (2) have upper GI disease; or (3) are taking oral anticoagulants. Reduces fever by direct action on hypothalamic heat-regulating centers, which increases dissipation of body heat via vasodilation and sweating.	*Adult:* 325-650 mg PO q6h, or 1000 mg tid/qid; not to exceed 4 g/d *Pediatric:* <12 years: 10-15 mg/kg/dose PO q4-6h prn; not to exceed 2.6 g/d >12 y: 650 mg q4h; not to exceed 5 doses in 24 h
Ibuprofen (Motrin®, Advil®, Nuprin®)	Drug of choice for treatment of mild to moderately severe pain, if no contraindications. Inhibits inflammatory reactions and pain, probably by decreasing activity of enzyme cyclooxygenase, in turn inhibiting prostaglandin synthesis. One of few NSAIDs indicated for reduction of fever.	*Adult:* 200-400 mg PO q4-6h while symptoms persist; not to exceed 3.2 g/d *Pediatric:* <16 y: 5-10 mg/kg/dose PO q6-8h prn; max: 50 mg/kg/day >16 y: Administer as in adults

Prognosis

Generally, the prognosis of herpes zoster oticus is good. However, in some cases, hearing loss may be permanent. Vertigo may last for days or weeks. Facial paralysis may be temporary or permanent.

The rash usually resolves within 14-21 days. Postherpetic neuralgia is defined as pain persisting at least 1 month after the rash has healed. Its incidence increases dramatically with age (i.e., 4% in those aged 30-50 years, 50% in those older than 80 years).

Vaccines—Elicit active immunization to increase resistance to infection. Vaccines consist of attenuated microorganisms or cellular components, which act as antigens. Administration stimulates antibody production with specific protective properties.		
Drug name	**Indication**	**Dosing**
Varicella zoster vaccine (Zostavax®)	Lyophilized preparation of Oka/Merck strain of live attenuated varicella-zoster virus. Shown to boost immunity against herpes zoster virus (shingles) in older patients. Reduces occurrence of shingles in individuals >60 y by about 50%. For individuals aged 60-69 y, it reduces occurrence by 64%. Also slightly reduces pain compared with no vaccination in those who develop shingles. Indicated for prevention of herpes zoster.	*Adult:* <60 y: Not established ≥60 y: Following reconstitution with entire vial of diluent supplied, use separate sterile needle and syringe to withdraw entire contents of reconstituted vial (0.65 ml) and administer subcutaneously X1 dose; administer in upper arm *Pediatric:* Not indicated.

Prevention

A new vaccine, marketed as Zostavax®, has been approved for persons 60 years of age or older with a history of chicken pox and with immunocompromise due to cancer, HIV, active tuberculosis, or chronic steroid use or other immunosuppressive medications. Only one injection is required and the cost is approximately $150.00. This vaccine reduces the chances of developing shingles by 51%. For those who develop shingles nonetheless, the severity of the disease is markedly ameliorated. The side effects of the vaccine are minor and include pain, tenderness, and swelling at the injection site. Some patients report mild headache.

Summary for Herpes Zoster Oticus

Herpes zoster oticus is a viral infection caused by varicella zoster, which initially produces chickenpox and can later result in shingles. If there is a reactivation of the varicella-zoster virus along the distribution of the sensory nerves innervating the ear, Ramsay Hunt syndrome occurs. Ramsay Hunt syndrome is a relatively common complication of shingles and accounts for up to 12% of all facial paralyses in the United States. Complications can be numerous, with postherpetic neuralgia the most common. Regarding treatment, most cases are self-limited and require only treatment of the symptoms with antiviral agents, corticosteroids, or analgesics. A new vaccine, Zostavax®, has been approved for persons 60 years or age or older and reduces the chances of developing shingles by 51%.

SKULL BASE OSTEOMYELITIS/MALIGNANT OTITIS EXTERNA/NECROTIZING OTITIS EXTERNA[3]

Skull base osteomyelitis is a potentially devastating infection. Osteomyelitis of the skull base, by definition, is an infection particularly within the diploic cancellous bone of the outer and/or inner cortical tables, the periosteum, dura, surrounding soft tissue, major vessels, and cranial nerves of the skull base. The most typical patient is an elderly, uncontrolled diabetic with pseudomonal infection and facial palsy.

Terminology

Skull base osteomyelitis is often referred to as "malignant otitis externa." The term "malignant" is used to emphasize the serious nature of this infection. Unfortunately, the term is misleading since there is no true "malignant" characteristic to the disease process, and some have called it a dangerous misnomer. Despite these misgivings, the term "malignant otitis externa" remained in common use in the literature. Patients hearing this diagnosis consistently confuse it with cancer. Such confusion by clinicians and patients alike prompted a search for other names. Various alternative terms used are progressive, fulminant, invasive, and necrotizing external otitis. The latter term, *necrotizing otitis externa,* is currently the most appropriate and widely accepted and has been offered as an alternative.

Signs and Symptoms

This condition should be suspected when, despite adequate topical treatment, otalgia and headache are disproportionately more severe than the clinical signs or when granulation tissue is apparent at the bony cartilaginous junction (Figure 6-7).

Skull base osteomyelitis follows a specific and direct pattern of anatomic spread beginning in the epithelium of the EAC and extending into the retromandibular fossa through the fissure of Santorini into the parotid space or through the tympanomastoid suture. Facial palsy is typically due to soft tissue infection around the stylomastoid foramen.

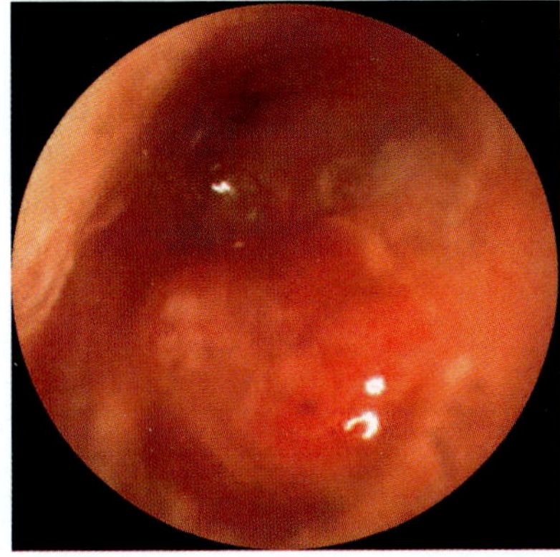

Figure 6-7. Necrotizing otitis externa. Here, the ear canal is moist, inflamed, and filled with granulation tissue.

In turn, the infection extends to the mastoid tip and jugular foramen. In some cases, thrombosis of the sigmoid sinus occurs with or without lower cranial nerve paresis or paralysis. Transvenous thrombosis may involve the lateral sinus and the superior and inferior petrosal sinuses. Dissemination of septic emboli may ensue. Progressive osteomyelitis further advances into the petrous apex, middle cranial fossa, base of the sphenoid, and clivus of the posterior cranial fossa. Contralateral temporal bone and skull base involvement is possible and has been reported. Posterior spread into the occipital bone elicits neural pain and potential compromise of the contents of the posterior cranial fossa. Rarely, extension anteriorly into the temporal fossa and facial bone may also occur.

Etiology

Waldrogel identified three fundamental factors that define the pathogenesis of the disease:

- A contiguous focus of infection
- Haematogenous seeding and
- Microvascular diseases

Known microvascular disease, complicating diabetes mellitus in elderly diabetics, and poor glucose control compromise blood supply to the affected area limiting effective host immunologic response and, in turn, host defense against the infection. Diabetes mellitus is the most common predisposing, co-morbid factor identified in 90% of patients. The majority of patients are aged 60 years or older.

Other predisposing factors are use of hearing aid, chronic suppurative otitis media, leukemia, alcoholism, kernicterus, tuberculosis, and frequent swimming. Rubin found in a retrospective study that 61.5% of patients underwent ear irrigation with unsterile tap water within 2 weeks of the onset of symptoms by their physicians.

Other than *Staphylococcus aureus* and *Staphylococcus epidermidis*, other less common organisms isolated in both adults and children are salmonella, *Mycobacterium tuberculosis*, Actionomyces, *Aspergillus flavus,* and *Aspergillus fumigatus.* In spite of a fairly long list of pathogens reported to have been isolated, it is important to keep in mind that *Pseudomonas* species are found in 99.2% of cases.

> **PDQ fact**: *Skull base osteomyelitis has grave morbidity and warrants a high degree of suspicion when formulating a differential diagnosis for otogenic skull base lesions.*

Diagnosis

Skull base osteomyelitis has grave morbidity and warrants a high degree of suspicion when formulating a differential diagnosis for otogenic skull base lesions. If untreated, it may extend throughout the skull base, infratemporal fossa, parapharyngeal space, and nasopharynx to extend intracranially.

Other diagnoses in the differential that may present along the skull base and with similar symptoms and signs are Wegener's granulomatosis, temporal bone carcinoma, nasopharyngeal carcinoma, metastatic lesion to the clivus, Paget's disease, fibrous dysplasia, and basilar skull fracture.

Notwithstanding the fact that there are no absolute diagnostic criteria, Cohen and Friedman developed diagnostic criteria classified as either obligatory or occasional. The major obligatory criteria include:

- Pain
- Exudate
- Edema
- Granulation tissue
- Microabscess
- Positive technitium-99 scan
- Failure of ototopical therapy after more than 1 week and
- The presence of *Pseudomonas aeruginosa*

The minor occasional criteria include positive CT scan, old age (50 years or older), cranial nerve palsy, diabetes mellitus, or other debilitating conditions. Contemporary head and neck neuroradiologists debate the need for radionucleotide studies and support CT scan as the sole imaging modality needed to make the diagnosis.

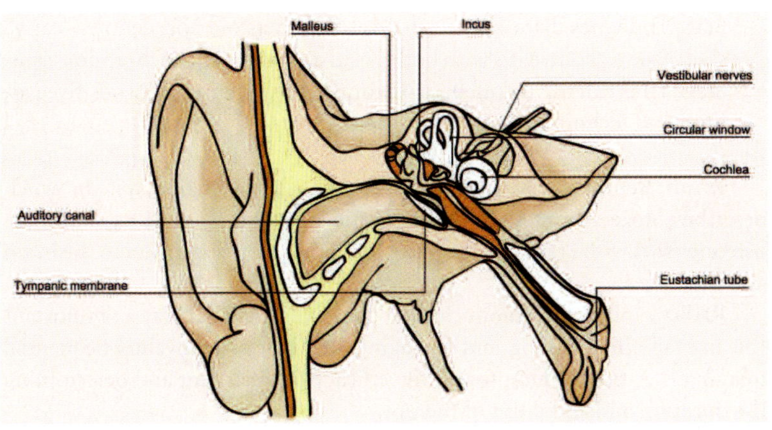

The role of MRI continues to be debated. In the absence of otologic complaints and findings, skull base osteomyelitis may be very difficult to diagnose. Isolated case reports have been published that review the condition without any history of OE. The clinician must be aware of any prior history of skull base osteomyelitis despite having received successful treatment, as these patients not uncommonly leave the hospital completely asymptomatic only to return 4 to 7 weeks later with the onset of low-grade fever, malaise, and a unilateral unremitting headache that requires narcotic analgesia. It has also been reported that skull base osteomyelitis can develop nearly 1 year after resolution of a more contained episode of necrotizing otitis externa.

Rare cases have been reported in children with *P. aeruginosa* and *Proteus mirabilis* OE. Furthermore, the condition associated with children are anemia, malnutrition, Stevens-Johnson Syndrome, immunoglobulin deficiency, and agranulocytosis. It is proposed that the more medial location of the bony cartilaginous junction in infants and children accounts for earlier involvement of the facial nerve and mastoid.

Staging and Imaging

The importance of staging is to alert the clinician that certain diagnostic tests are necessary to determine the presence and extent of the disease. Gallium-67 scanning identifies inflammation if immunocompetent white cells are present and functioning. The technitium-99 bone scan reflects the increased osteoblastic activity, which is indicative of osteitis and osteomyelitis. Benecke proposed a three-level staging:

- Stage I is deeply invasive infection limited to the soft tissue without bone involvement.

- Stage II defines disease that extends to the mastoid and denotes "early" skull base osteomyelitis with both positive gallium and technitium scans.
- Stage III is extensive skull base osteomyelitis with markedly positive gallium and technitium scan.

Krum, Rehm, and Kenny have proposed a third staging system, which describes Stage I limited to the EAC and mastoid, Stage II as skull base osteomyelitis with cranial nerve palsy, and Stage III as extension to the brain and meninges.

Radiographic and radionucleide including Indium-III play an important role in evaluating, staging, and managing skull base osteomyelitis. Sequential imaging is critical in monitoring the efficacy of treatment and determining the duration and end point of therapy.

Treatment

Skull base osteomyelitis is difficult to treat, and the mortality rate can be as high as 53%. The complex management of the condition begins with correctly establishing the diagnosis, determining the extent of the disease, providing appropriate antimicrobial therapy along with adjuvant therapy, and operating when indicated. Underlying metabolic abnormalities must be identified and corrected. Particularly, tight blood sugar control must be maintained.

PDQ fact: *Although many antibiotic regimens have been proposed, prolonged antibiotic therapy with third-generation cephalosporins has been the principal means of therapy for skull base osteomyelitis.*

Antibiotic Management

Although many antibiotic regimens have been proposed, prolonged antibiotic therapy with third-generation cephalosporins has been the principal means of therapy. A combination of a beta-lactam antibiotic and aminoglycoside has also been effective. Management has significantly evolved in the last decade in the wake of oral fluoroquinolones such as ciprofloxacin. In a report by Rubin, patients were cured using a combination of ciprofloxacin and rifampicin for 6 to 12 weeks. Oral ciprofloxacin alone in 750 mg BID dose cured 21 out of 23 patients treated by Lang. Surprisingly, ciprofloxacin given orally for a minimum of 6 weeks and for as long as 6 months was successful in patients who failed conventional combination intravenous therapy. The excellent gastrointestinal absorption of the fluoroquinolones allows milder infections to be treated with a 2-week course of oral therapy.

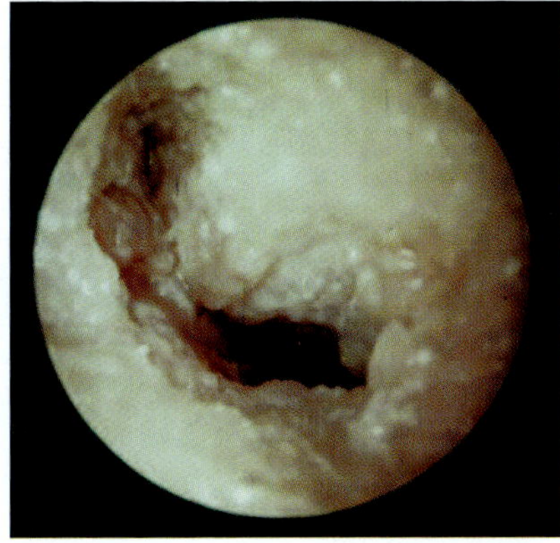

Squamous cell carcinoma. No otoscopic signs are truly diagnostic of malignant tumors of the external auditory canal. The most suspicious symptoms are bleeding from the external canal and chronic otorrhoea that has recently become associated with pain. When pain or bleeding develops in cases of chronic otitis externa or chronic suppurative otitis media, a careful inspection of the ear must be carried out to exclude the possibility of an underlying neoplasm. Any unusual or uncharacteristic growths arising in the external canal must have a biopsy.

Similar efficacy with ofloxacin (200 mg) dosed BID in 17 patients achieved subjective improvement in all patients within 6 days and objective improvement within 12 days of treatment.

Despite the reported efficacy of prolonged systemic antibiotic therapy, treatment failures do occur.

Adjunctive Medical Therapy

The most likely mechanism underlying treatment failure when culture-directed antibiotics have been chosen on the basis of *in vitro* susceptibility testing is tissue hypoperfusion and hypoxia. In such cases, hyperbaric oxygen, which increases wound PO_2 levels, enhances phagocytic oxidative killing of aerobic micro-organisms, and promotes angioneogenesis and osteoneogenesis, should be strongly considered. Treatment consists of 100% O_2 given for 90 minutes at 2.5 atmospheres of absolute pressure 5 days a week for a total duration of treatment of 4 weeks as an adjuvant therapy.

Surgery

Surgery is rarely required but may be necessary in cases where devitalized sequestrations of bone may need to be debrided. The role of surgery is by and large adjunctive to mainstay medical therapy but has a role for diagnostic biopsy in addition to local debridement of necrotic tissue already mentioned. Finally, surgery may also be important to drain abscesses.

The specific operation is tailored to the clinical picture and may include formal tympanomastoidectomy as a modified or radical canal wall down mastoidectomy with or without partial petrous apicectomy and embolectomy when septic jugular vein thrombosis is present. Farrier proposed planned surgical debridement for persistent pain or failure of granulation tissue to resolve after 2 weeks of intravenous antibiotics. Raines and Schindler advocated radical surgery in the face of new onset cranial neuropathies. Concern exists that surgery may actually worsen prognosis by creating iatrogenic facial spaces and new tissue planes allowing even further spread of the infection.

Following Treatment Response

A combination of technetium scanning to detect osteoblastic activity and gallium 67 imaging to detect granulocytic activity is recommended by some as a means of monitoring response to treatment. The erythrocyte sedimentation rate can also be used to monitor therapeutic response.

Complications and Prognosis

Cranial nerve neuropathy is the most common non-iatrogenic complication. *P. aeruginosa* elaborates destructive enzymes and exotoxins that promote tissue necrosis and reversible neurotoxicity. Other than facial palsy, the jugular foramen syndrome involving cranial nerves 9, 10, and 11 affects phonation, swallowing, and protection of the lower airway. Other cranial nerves that may be affected are the oculomotor, trigeminal, and abducens nerve. In untreated or advanced cases, death may result due to meningitis, cerebritis, cerebral abscess, jugular foramen syndrome, pulmonary aspiration and pneumonia, vascular thrombosis, stroke, or subarachnoid hemorrhage. The mortality rate is high when multiple cranial neuropathies occur despite optimal antimicrobial therapy. Recent reports with appropriate antibiotic therapy, however, estimate cure rates at 80-100%. Use of hyperbaric O_2 as an adjuvant therapy has also further reduced the mortality rate.

Summary for Skull Base Osteomyelitis

Skull base osteomyelitis is an aggressive, invasive, and often indolent infection with potentially significant morbidity and mortality. The most common form is seen in elderly diabetics although infections may result from other neurosurgical and cranial base sources or procedures. The diagnosis is based on a detailed history, complete physical examination, culture, biopsy, blood sugar and metabolic measures, erythrocyte sedimentation rate, and imaging studies. Intravenous or oral anti-pseudomonal antibiotic therapy, surgical debridement of granulation tissue, bony sequestration and devitalized tissue from the EAC and skull base can control and cure the disease effectively. Treatment for recalcitrant infections should include adjuvant hyperbaric oxygen therapy. The course of antibiotic therapy varies from a short 2 to 3 weeks for stage I disease in children to 6 months for advanced cases in adults. The duration of therapy is determined by a number of factors including symptomatic and clinical response and demonstration of the resolution of inflammation by monitoring treatment with sequential CT scan, gallium scan, and erythrocyte sedimentation rate. The overall morbidity and mortality have significantly declined with current methods of diagnosis and treatment during the past three decades.

---

[1] Adapted from: http://www.emedicine/com/derm/topic193.htm

[2] Adapted from http://www.emedicine.com/EMERG/topic823.htm

[3] Adapted from: http://cyberlectures.indmedica.com/show/96/1/Malignant%20Otitis%20Externa

Case Studies

CASE 1

A 35-year-old otherwise healthy white male presents with a 2-day history of severe otalgia of the left ear, scant discharge, and "muffled hearing." The patient had been training for an upcoming triathalon, which included daily swimming. The patient had no known drug allergies, had never had surgery, and was in excellent health prior to the onset of symptoms.

Physical examination revealed a healthy-appearing male with normal vital signs and without fever. Extreme tenderness was elicited upon attempted manipulation of the auricle. The ear canal was diffusely edematous and a "cheesy" exudate was seen throughout the canal. Although erythematous, the tympanic membrane was visualized and mobile upon examination with pneumatic otoscopy. No spread beyond the confines of the external auditory canal was seen and the remainder of the physical examination was normal.

A working diagnosis of diffuse acute otitis externa was made and the patient was placed on topical neomycin/polymyxin B/hydrocortisone (Cortisporin® Otic). Ibuprofen was recommended for pain management and the patient was advised to stop swimming and to observe dry ear precautions when bathing. At 1 week, the patient continued to complain of severe pruritus and discharge. Examination continued to reveal significant inflammation of the external auditory canal and 2 additional weeks of Cortisporin® Otic was advised. After 3 days, the patient called and stated that his symptoms were worse and that now the outer ear was red. Repeat evaluation confirmed a cellulitis of the pinna and an orally administered, first-generation cephalosporin was added. There was no improvement after 48 hours of both the topical and systemic antibiotic. The patient was referred to an otolaryngologist. The impression was that of allergy to the neomycin. All medications were stopped and the patient significantly improved. Follow-up examination 2 weeks later revealed resolution of the inflammation but no cerumen production was seen. Topical acetic acid was used after all water exposures until normal cerumen production resumed after which all treatments were discontinued and the patient discharged from specialty care.

CASE 2

A 3-year-old female presented to her pediatrician with a 3-day history of right ear pain. She had no fever but was very irritable and sleeping poorly. The child was in daycare and had "continuous" nasal congestion. The family had just returned from a weekend at their lake house and the child had been swimming in the baby pool while there.

The child's past medical history, family history, and social history were otherwise normal.

On physical examination, the child was afrebile with an oral temperature of 37.5 degrees Celsuis. Her respiratory rate was 20 and unlabored. Her pulse was 118 beats per minute and regular. She was normotensive. Her right ear canal was quite edematous and there was postauricular edema and protrusion of the lobule as per the photographs below.

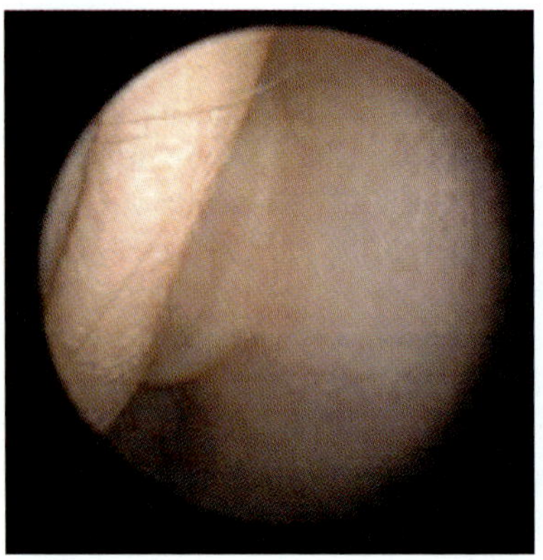 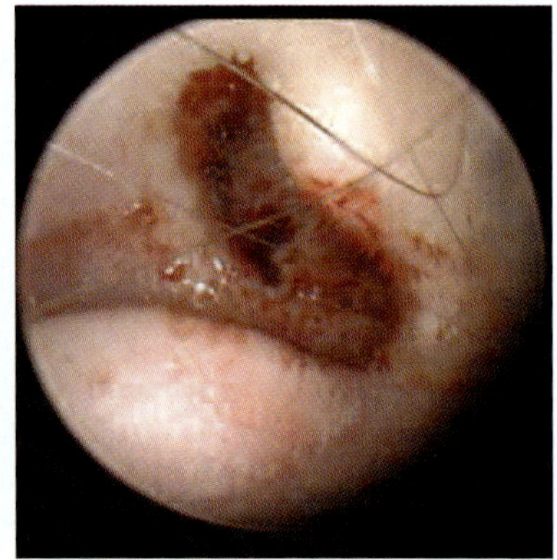

The remainder of the examination was normal except for bilateral mucoid rhinorrhea. The diagnosis of otitis externa was made and the child was treated with Ciprodex® Otic and, because of extension of the acute otitis externa beyond the confines of the external auditory canal, Keflex® was added. Unfortunately, the child's condition worsened and she was reassessed 3 days later. There was markedly less swelling of the ear canal on examination, likely due to the ciprofloxacin/dexamethasone treatment and the tympanic membrane was fully visualized. It is shown below.

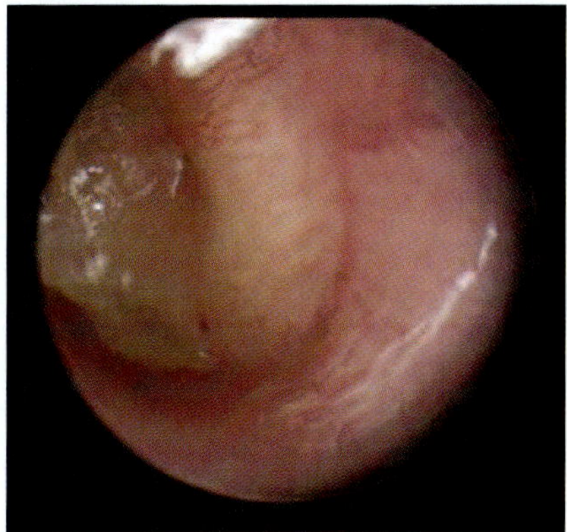

The child's diagnosis was now acute otitis media with secondary otitis externa and at this point it was unclear as to whether the postauricular edema represented an extension of the otitis externa or acute coalescent mastoiditis. A CT scan was obtained.

There was no evidence of acute coalescent mastoiditis and, based on the patient's past history or recurrent acute otitis media, the decision was made to take the patient to the operating room and perform bilateral myringotomy with tympanostomy tubes. At the time of surgery, purulent middle-ear effusions were sampled and *S. pneumonia*, demonstrating intermediate resistance to penicillin, was isolated. The child was treated post-operatively with oral amoxicillin/clavulanic acid and topical ciprofloxacin/dexamethasone and was completely recovered in 3 days.

Index

P

R

S